Auto-Immune Disease & Fibromyalgia:

The Traumatic Brain Injury Connection

C. Rae Johnson

Copyright

Information within this book is for educational purposes only. It
is not intended to replace your physician or medical care. Please
see your health-care provider before beginning suggestions in
this book or any new health program; for complete well-being.

ISBN: 978-1-387-91516-3

Dedication

This book is dedicated for the Glory of God Alone. To my Lord and all His children who are suffering through the effects of brain injuries and the aftermath that follows; auto-immune disorders and Fibromyalgia. It is only through His peace, comfort, love, mercy, grace and strength that we are ultimately able to continue on forward, joyfully in the hopes of helping others get through their pain.

Soli Deo Gloria

Glory to God Alone

Acknowledgments

I just want to acknowledge with a heartfelt thank you to my family for allowing me the time to accomplish another feat in writing another book; something I thought I would be unable to do, due to having a brain injury along with the health struggles I am still experiencing as a direct result. But God is good! I love you all! Enjoy!

I also would like to thank my husband John for his clever cover design and willingness to put up with me in going the extra mile in making it perfect; as tedious as it may be. Thanks Babe!

I would also very much like to acknowledge my appreciation to Matt Dahl, creator, trainer and CEO of the Sanddune Stepper rehabilitation training tool, who was so thoughtful and kind enough to send me my very own. Matt, I appreciate you and your input with much advice along with the timely help, more than you will ever know. God Bless you brother. You are touching and changing lives for the better!

Auto-Immune Disease

&

Fibromyalgia:

The

Traumatic Brain Injury Connection

Contents

Introduction

Okay, here we go, with yet another brain book. You may be wondering, "What more can be discussed?" The answer is plenty! The begging question that is answered, is in the aftermath or fall-out that so many people, including doctors, "miss" yet is fully experienced from the point of onset of a Traumatic Brain Injury and well past, by the one going through it.

Through my own personal experiences of having a Traumatic Brain Injury, over 4 years ago to the writing of this book, I have also had the privilege of experiencing a lengthy Post-Concussion Syndrome, and still do struggle a bit with proprioception issues as well as light, sound and smell intolerances, in addition to memory challenges. I am also privy to what so often comes next. I am currently in the next phase of injury that no one talks about, nor informs you about; perhaps due to the unknowing of the connection.

I've had the continual blood work to stump doctors in awe of what is taking place. I experience daily the ongoing "new" symptoms to only add to the never-ending puzzle. I've been diagnosed with a different auto-immune disease every time I go to the specialist's office, only to walk out with no definitive answer. It's always a "maybe this", or "maybe that".

Now I finally have more of an answer as it is getting narrowed down to at least include Fibromyalgia; and boy do I have the symptoms of experience. It is a ride for sure; but one that is promising that I can get some relief and eventually get off the ride. So, can you!

When we continue to go to our doctor's office, and though most really do want to help, they almost seem unable as they are perplexed at the new cascade of oncoming symptoms, only to refer us to other specialists, blood work and more tests. Our blood work may reveal eye opening glimpses of what is going on in our bodies that is enough to place a fright within us. Our specialists may offer solutions of prescription drugs, only to find we are no better off, because then what surfaces are even more health concerns. "What the heck happened?" we wonder as we are more bewildered than ever. "Can our lives ever, ever, get back to normal again?" By the way, what is normal as most of us had forgotten the sweet smell of normalcy.

Fret not! Don't you know that no one is normal anyway? We are actually well beyond normal or even just ordinary for all what we have been through. In fact, we just happen to be "extra"ordinary! That's a good thing! Hmmmm....Just think for a moment that you are indeed extraordinary and you will get through this. I promise! Look, if I can do it, anyone can. You can do this. We are only given what we can handle, so you must be able to handle this, and then perhaps even help others going through the same thing one day. This is not the end, again like we once thought when we first suffered a brain injury. This is just another chapter in "your" book called life. What you will find in this book are hopefully helpful tips and advice to combat the many woes of health concerns, while making educated and wise choices for a better future; and that future, starts today!

For I know the plans I have for you," declares the LORD, "plans to prosper you and not to harm you, plans to give you hope and a future. Jeremiah 29:11NIV

Damaged Brain + Adrenal Fatigue = Disease

Okay, so you had a Traumatic Brain Injury and have been struggling with Post-Concussion Syndrome; perhaps for some time now. Now what? You've been to the doctor's office, more of them then you care to count or travel to, possibly due to lingering symptoms. The answers overall to your plight seem the same with little to no difference in diagnosis. The overall concluding diagnosis that anyone who is still struggling hates to hear is that, "It's just anxiety" or "A concussion heals in two weeks", or even "It's all in your head". Well yeah, in a way it is; "It's called a brain injury doc and my brain is in my head", you long to reply.

So, what is going on? Well, damage does not stop at the point of impact. In fact, it has a ripple effect, much like a butterfly effect; and the point of impact, the initial traumatic brain injury, is only the beginning. Sadly, many doctors, neurologists even, think we are healed in two weeks. Not so! The patient knows.

A blow to the head, a quick jolt, a sudden movement, all causing a concussion, even lack of oxygen to the brain as a result of a brain injury or surgery can result in a Traumatic Brain Injury (TBI for short). According to the CDC (Centers for Disease,

Control and Prevention) it is estimated that there are 1.7 million new cases of TBI"s each year; and those are just the ones reported. Out of that number there are 52,000 deaths, 275,000 hospitalizations, and 1,365,000 emergency room visits with 80% of those cases being treated and released. That is astounding!

Out of these cases of patients who are just released often find themselves at a loss as to what has not only happened to them but is continually happening as their symptoms do not go away but only linger as new ones are developed and noticed through activities of daily living. Many in turn develop what is known as Post-Concussion Syndrome (PCS for short). There is a loss of not only productivity within one's life including family and careers, but also the medical costs can be staggering, estimating 60 Billion in the United States alone, as individuals search for effective solutions to help with daily living.

Why is it that medically trained professionals, many of them neurologists mind you, (specialists in the field of neurology—a branch of medicine dealing with disorders of the nervous system) who see so many patients with concussions, blow them off as if they are psychiatric in nature rather then injury related presenting with real damage to the brain and nervous system? It is just mind boggling even for the intact brain injury free individual. These are real live people with their lives being impacted in every imaginable way due to a brain injury and yet, they are so easily dismissed. I finally, after several neurologists, found one that is very conscientious and is checking everything including nerve damage. He is not overlooking any symptom. He is a doctor truly wanting to help his patients, as is my family doctor. After all, isn't that what they ultimately went to school for, to help people?

A reason for some doctors not being as helpful, can be a lack of knowledge on the physician's part along with lack of empathy; unless they have personally gone through it within their own lives or in that of their family.

Sometimes, and I say this lightly because it is actually many times and probably most times, a concussion does not heal within two weeks and if there is damage within the brain causing a disconnect throughout the body, Post-Concussion Syndrome is then prevalent and long-lasting.

When Post-Concussion Syndrome lasts longer than expected or what is originally told by a physician, it can become troublesome and very much confusing and disheartening as we can no longer function quite as we did prior to the injury; and we cannot tell when we will ever be able to again. It becomes a sort of big obstacle, a giant in our way of life. We are faced with lifestyle changes that must be made in order to function on a daily basis. We find that we are off balance still when we are in unfamiliar surroundings. The sights, smells and sounds still really bug us and send us off into a tizzy of internal disruption that ripples outwardly into our immediate surroundings. We find that we have to get away immediately from that noise, such as a twangy guitar, violin, or any high-pitched sounds or chatter from a group of people talking, as we cover our ears in desperation.

The unpleasant smells that somehow send a direct offensive signal to the brain make us feel as though we are suddenly suffocating in a poisonous gas. The sights we see can go from a serene calm to an immediate storm as an influx of visual displays overload our seemingly simple mind; though it be quite complex to deal with and decipher all that is bombarding it on a continuous basis. We then instantly and even somehow unexpectantly hit a wall of weaponry that is bent on attack to our nervous system, an arsenal that is otherwise benign to an uninjured, uncompromised individual. Straightaway people, including doctors, often view us as unstable or even coo-coo just because they are not experiencing the same overwhelming brain overload that we are. No wonder they are quick to judge and label it all as "just anxiety".

When these overloads happen, they affect the body in other ways as well, for instance our speech may slow remarkably as we are also tipsy in our gate; making us to seem to be under an alcohol or drug induced state of being. Our blood pressure and pulse may rise significantly, causing more dizziness and other physiological concerns, mimicking heart problems prompting the use of blood pressure medication. Other physiological functions in the body may soon be noticed as the disconnect from the brain to the body is allowed to continue unnoticed. There will be a strain on the adrenal glands (endocrine glands—endocrine system) which are responsible for hormone production in the body, in adequate and correct amounts to maintain health or homeostasis; a stable equilibrium for normal bodily functioning without disease.

Now when there is a disturbance within the body, there is a disturbance in the force, your overall health and functioning. Strange symptoms start popping up that can be so numerous as to confuse most medical professionals, because they want to treat the symptoms...not the cause! If what a person, a patient, is exhibiting upon a physical exam, mimics obvious symptoms, that is what they will most likely treat. Anxiety-like symptoms are going to be treated with prescribed anti-anxiety meds, and therefore will be labeled psychiatric in nature, that will also be in your medical record.

Therefore, once a person starts a medication, whether it be a psychiatric drug or even a blood pressure pill, it will be much harder for them to get off of them but only to find they may experience new problems, new symptoms, relating to the medication they have been prescribed. Have they gotten any better? Most likely no, because the underlying cause has not been treated. All they received was a band-aid for a gaping hole. All this can lead to a state of downcast moods and even depression, to the point that many doctors will only want to further prescribe pharmaceutical medication in a downward spiral. But it does not have to be this way. Once we begin to really understand what is taking place within our body and brain, learning about the root causes and how to affectively deal with them and treat them, we can improve.

The internal environment of the body is still very much compromised and undergoing a great deal of stress. There is an ongoing inflammatory process taking place that is now flowing throughout the body, no longer just at the site of impact where the inflammation from the original injury impact occurred. The stage is set. The bodily systems are not relating to each other, nor to the brain. There is a disconnect due to damage; damage of the lobes causing a host of symptoms relating to each particular lobe and their unique function within the body.

There is damage to the neurons and axons making communication not only difficult or incomplete, but also many times completely gone; severed, for the time being at least. If there is damage to the hypothalamus and pituitary gland, then there are incorrect amounts of hormones being produced as well as inhibited. The hormones produced in the pituitary gland help regulate the overall functions of the endocrine system, which has an effect on the production of key hormones such as reproductive hormones, steroidal hormones as in cortisol (stress hormone), and growth hormones affecting metabolism.

Prolactin, otherwise known as luteotropic hormone, is a protein not only responsible for its role in milk production in females but is also dominant in affecting other essential processes of the human body including metabolism, pancreatic development and regulating the immune system. Prolactin is secreted by the pituitary gland in response to such things as eating, mating, ovulating and nursing as well as estrogen therapy treatment. The prolactin secretion in the pituitary gland is regulated by endocrine neurons in the hypothalamus.

If there is damage to one or both, either the hypothalamus or the pituitary gland then communication is altered and therefore causes an imbalance as it will not only have an effect on hormones but also on the regulation of blood clotting and dopamine secretion, (a neurotransmitter released by neurons, sending signals to other nerves). Now Dopamine, produced by the hypothalamus, is however one of the main regulators in the production of Prolactin, within the pituitary gland. Dopamine is responsible for restraining prolactin production, so the more dopamine, the less prolactin is released. Prolactin then will enhance the secretion of dopamine. I know, this is confusing! Think of it as a feedback loop, a negative feedback loop of a slowing down process.

Negative and positive feedback loops are a slowing down and an accelerating process of producing, releasing and restraining necessary components to a healthy life; in this case, proteins, hormones, and neurotransmitters all affected by amino acids, enzymes and injury. Our bodies are in such precise alignment with each tiny, infinitely microscopic cell, protein molecule, enzyme and so forth, that our homeostasis is capable of great things such as keeping us functioning properly while our bodies heal and grow. The human body is truly amazing; and we are truly fearfully and wonderfully made.

I don't mean to confuse you even further but there is another important and main regulator of prolactin that not only increases the production but also the secretion of prolactin within the pituitary gland. That regulator, that hormone is estrogen. Now, it is important for the female body to have an increase of prolactin at times in their reproductive cycle (during pregnancy) and after giving birth; for the very reason of lactation (milk production) to prepare the body to feed a newborn baby. There are other hormones as well that do have an impact on the production of prolactin but these two discussed here have a great impact on the body, not only in terms of how much prolactin is floating around but also, they by themselves with either too little or too much can have a negative impact, resulting in bodily system dysfunction. We'll discuss more in the next chapter on the impact and strain to the adrenal glands caused by incorrect amounts of hormones in the body.

Dopamine pathways are involved with releasing hormones as well as motor control. It is said to bring about desire and pleasure, therefore with an imbalance or lack, depression-like symptoms and melancholy moods are more pronounced. Dopamine also functions as a vasodilator and inhibits norepinephrine release. It also helps the kidneys to excrete sodium in urine, helps the digestive system by reducing gastrointestinal motility and protecting the intestinal mucosa, reduces insulin production in the pancreas, and is also known to modulate immune function regulating the activity of lymphocytes (white blood cells—natural killer cells T and B) in the immune system; protecting your body from a foreign invader.

When there is dysfunction in neural communication and a loss of dopamine secreting neurons, a degenerative disease such as Parkinson's can take place, causing motor impairment and tremors. Not only so, but decreased dopamine activity is also associated with ADHD (Attention Deficit Hyperactivity Disorder) as well as Restless Leg Syndrome (often accompanies Fibromyalgia), and if anyone needs to take a antipsychotic medication for such conditions as schizophrenia, they are most likely treated with a dopamine antagonist which reduces dopamine activity further.

Dopamine is a key neurotransmitter and also a precursor to other neurotransmitters and hormones such as Epinephrine (adrenaline), which is secreted by the adrenal glands mainly and has a direct impact on the heart by increasing cardiac output. It also impacts blood glucose levels and prepares a person for a "fight-or-flight" mode when under stress. Dopamine, though found in many food sources such as eggs, omega-3 rich fish, bananas, almonds, walnuts, dark chocolate, dairy and unprocessed meats, does not however cross the blood/brain barrier that protects the brain. Therefore, it needs to be synthesized inside the brain to be able to perform its synaptic transmission as a neurotransmitter. Because Dopamine is synthesized within the neurons of the brain and also in cells of the adrenal glands, it requires the correct amount of both essential (not made by the body but comes from food) and non-essential (made-synthesized within the body) amino acids to synthesize, as well as enzymes that are essential for conversion throughout the process.

As you can see there is a ripple effect of a disruption of key neurotransmitters and hormone production within the body and how levels can be altered, just through injury, that affects more key secretions, causing a wide array of negative effects within the human body and within the many bodily systems. It all starts with something and in this case, a brain injury; enough to label it a Traumatic Brain Injury (TBI) signifying "trauma" directly to the brain. Trauma means damage to tissues, nerves, cells, et cetera, as everything is impacted. There is a huge inflammatory process started and it does not just go away in two weeks. A big healing process is also underway as the body fights to hold it all together; an operation to run efficiently and effectively while protecting itself from further damage. When wrong levels of key components are made and secreted, there is chaos within; disharmony and lack of homeostasis.

Prolactin directly secreted by the Pituitary gland is a necessary component, critical key hormone and protein, that has an effect branching outwardly within the systems via neurotransmitters, impacting the adrenal glands, and quite possibly setting the stage for disease and an impaired immune function; the beginning stages of an auto-immune disease/disorder. Every and any brain injury should be taken very seriously, because it is very serious, and the effects have the possibility of being detrimental for the body, for the person who is going through the whole process.

A brain injured individual should have a caring and conscientious doctor that will take the time to listen, to really listen to what is going on and to consider all the symptoms being experienced, no matter how little they are or seemingly insignificant they may sound, and also perhaps similar to or mimicking other health issues that are not really related. An MRI should be done as well as blood work including a reproductive hormonal panel along with thyroid function tests to monitor and check for imbalances along with any vitamin D deficiency. We need to know if indeed there is damage to the hypothalamus, to the Pituitary Gland, and to the Adrenal Glands. We want to avoid adrenal fatigue and stop it as soon as it starts. We want to get the body back to a state of healthiness, back to homeostasis. For that, we need to keep monitoring at least every 6 months, sooner if any different or new symptoms appear.

Additionally, we should get chiropractic care to fix any misalignments within our spinal cord or neck, that connects to the brain. If there is compression of nerves that run along the spinal column, or injury undetected such as bulging disks, that can pose a problem in our healing process by creating new ones if nerves are being further damaged, it can affect our entire nervous system. The brain is the control center of the body and the spinal column is the highway to every part of the body. It must be clear of injurious debris. It is far better to get to the heart of the problem before new ones are created. Why treat only the symptoms and not the underlying cause? That is the question we should all ask!

Beloved, I pray that in all respects you may prosper and be in good health, just as your soul prospers.
3 John 1:2 NASB

Heal me, O LORD, and I will be healed; Save me and I will be saved, For You are my praise.
Jeremiah 17:14 NASB

'Behold, I will bring to it health and healing, and I will heal them; and I will reveal to them an abundance of peace and truth.
Jeremiah 33:6 NASB

I call out to the LORD, and he answers me from his holy mountain.
Psalm 3:4 NIV

Auto-Immune Disease

You're getting out of bed and notice stiffness and pain in your feet. It starts off slowly, so you dismiss it as "over doing it" the day before. But, it keeps happening, enough so you start taking more notice. Then your family, friends or co-workers start to notice your movements as being somewhat impaired. You feel much stiffer all over and your hands and fingers start to ache and may even swell. The kids want to play, family and/or friends want to engage you in activities and projects, above and beyond what you may even have planned for yourself to be involved in and accomplish. However, that fatigue is back with a vengeance that is reminiscent of the beginning stages of your brain injury. You make yet another appointment at your doctor's office who runs some blood work and finds you have levels suggesting an auto-immune disease.

Somewhat shocked and slightly fearful you wonder what is next. Then a person says to you, "Wow your cheeks are so rosy and red! What shade of blush do you wear?" Funny thing is, you can't even remember the last time you wore blush, so you cleverly respond back in your wit, as you begin to lose your wits, "Oh thank you. It is a lovely shade of auto-immune!" The response on their face either makes you feel elated with your new-found humor, or about to cry thinking,

"Yep!" You scurry off to find a mirror to check your new rosiness and try to understand and accept your blossoming ruddy complexion. Hey, at least you don't need blush when applying make-up, even if you thought about it.

Adapting

Along with the new challenges of learning how to handle and adapt to an auto-immune disease also comes the pain of it all, with much focus on joints and some bone along with plenty of fatigue—ugh! Boy, the fatigue can be intense. You know what I'm talking about. You start off your day, first of all thankful you're alive, get out of bed and then start planning. You have, well, some energy, enough so you think to take on at least part of your day. That is until you start to do something, then suddenly, you're wiped out. But from what? It just feels like you were sidelined, and someone stole any ounce of energy you had. In return you received a whole lot of fatigue to the point of even thinking about doing something, just drains you.

"What in the world happened?" "How did I get here?" We often wonder. Most likely we will not even realize what could have set this off—this time bomb of an auto-immune disease/disorder. Personally, I prefer "disorder" rather than disease because disorder sounds more reversible and disease sounds, well, like the worst, like death. I don't want to be labeled with a death signal—I'm alive still. How about you? We just have to reverse the order, of the chaos. We may not be able to completely reverse everything in every case but with the right holistic approach and help from holistic minded doctors and therapy tools, we sure can feel a lot better. We can function more normally; if anything is even considered "normal" these days. But, if it's even close to normal, I'll take it. How about you? I don't want to be a victim with the "woe is me" claim. No, I want to be the best and feel the best I possibly can each and every day, with this gift we call life.

So, how did we get here? Oh yeah, that brain injury thing again. Geesh! "How much more damage can it cause?" We may wonder. It is the gift that can have the potential to keep on giving, even when we don't want it.

Now we had a brain injury, excuse me, a Traumatic Brain Injury. Yeah, that's more like it. Well, that "trauma" is still going on in the body if we are still struggling with symptoms and even sometimes when we don't know that we are. We may even feel fine, be completely cleared from our Doc and are just trying to get on with life; to finally move forward again. Then one day we go to the Doc and perhaps have some blood work. We may tell them upon our examination that, "Yeah, I am feeling a little fatigued lately, and sore too." We may notice it being harder and harder to get out of bed. When we place our feet on the floor, we may stumble a bit once we start to walk, from the uncomfortableness felt within them. We may feel stiff, like old age is setting in—just ignore I said that! I did not just say "old age"! After all, old age is relative. We are only as old as we feel or think we are, no matter how old we actually are.

But that Doc, well somehow may present to us age related health issues, even if we're young. Okay, something's going on here. If I'm young, why am I presenting with "arthritis" symptoms and walk and feel as though I'm older?

Okay, I've said it! That word. Arthritis. Actually, arthritis can affect the very young as we are starting to see more cases of it. So, what is going on here?

Well, our diets are not as healthy as before because many are not eating whole foods but in place of them are eating heavily processed foods with many chemical ingredients combining with unhealthy additives causing inflammation within the body, and the wholefoods that many of us do eat have been tampered with through genetic manipulation. Our air quality has also suffered from industries both current and from years past and so in these instances, changes happen within our bodies on a cellular level. We may have been exposed to other toxins, heavy metals, insecticides, molds, fungus and even parasites; not to mention a great deal of stress via our lifestyles which could be presenting us with numerous causes, anything from financial, marital, relational, occupational, emotional and now, more physical, as if a brain injury wasn't enough. Now some arthritis can be genetic by nature as say a parent or grandparent may have suffered from the same we may be dealing with—but many are not.

Through having an injury, inflammation is caused and especially having an injury to the brain, which is the control center of our bodies by way of the central and peripheral nervous systems, we have a problem. The inflammatory process going on caused by a Traumatic Brain Injury is absolutely huge. It deserves the phrase, "Houston, we have a problem!" In our case, "Body, we have a problem!" Add to that big inflammatory process an inflammatory diet with other environmental inflammatory stressors, including anything that increases our cortisol levels from living in stressful circumstance and we have the recipe for disaster and chaos within a calm and proficient environment. The inflammation takes our bodies over in an attempt to conquer.

We begin with inflammation in the brain as tissue has been injured, swelling has begun, neurons have been severed and axons have been stretched. The rest of our body is just trying to function as normal as possible, sending signals to the brain for help via the nervous system. But, there seems to be a disconnect and the signals are not getting through. Meanwhile we experience all kinds of symptoms and everything seems to be bothering us which only brings on more symptoms. The call is made again to the control center, the brain. But something's wrong. Things are not working properly as they have before.

We notice imbalances in our standing and gait as we attempt to even walk. We're suddenly tipping over, everywhere, hugging walls and feel as though we are "way off", tripping over our own feet, as others may think we're just drunk or drugged. We hear them speak and see their looks but we're having trouble responding. We notice we can't speak like we did before. We're stuttering and can't quite pronounce the word we want to use as we are attempting to pull it from some huge file within our brain, knowing that it's there, but we just can't find it. We can't even write as we normally can. We may feel lightheaded and dizzy, and the floor may even look all jumbled. We're caught in a crazy situation or some kind of bad dream.

Our proprioception may be well off and we may feel like we can't do anything. Our smell may have either left us or the exact opposite, which can lead to an overload quickly in the brain as we may not be able to stand certain smells because suddenly they are way too strong. We may become super sensitive in every respect, both our perceptions as well as our emotions. We may suddenly start to cry and not even know why, as others ask us, "What the heck is wrong with you?" We may start to feel like we're going crazy especially when loved ones and friends are not compassionate but rather react coldly in their fear of what they are witnessing in us. Doctors may not have the answers and dismiss almost every case as having an anxiety attack. But, we know better. We know that it is so much more. Anxiety, if we have it, is just the outcome from the bombarding stressors hitting everything that makes us, "us".

Physiologically, our blood pressure may rise along with our pulse. We find ourselves in fight-or-flight circumstances over virtually nothing. Our bodies go into survival mode and shut down what we do not need at that moment of intensity. It may shut down our speech and thought processes as we slow in the ability to even talk and think. We may have such memory problems that can make life a little dangerous as we constantly forget the stove is on—do not walk away. Even if we think we will remember, somehow, something else gets our attention as there is stimuli everywhere and we forget. We may have portions of memory just gone but somehow get stuck on repeating the same thing over and over again, as to not forget.

Our hormones start to fluctuate in response to the disconnect in the brain and nothing seems to be manufactured in the right amounts anymore as well as distributed in the correct amounts. Great fatigue may set in and we can't even begin to explain why; because we haven't done anything. All it takes is to "think" about doing something and we're already spent. Again, we tell the doctor what's going on, what we are experiencing but may be met with a response that suggests we just need more sleep.

Then unusual sensations of pain, stiffness and tingling may begin. We may still experience brain fog and slowness of thought so our new symptoms may even be dismissed by us ourselves. But they keep happening, almost everyday with some days being worse than others. Blood testing is finally taken with a host of abnormalities showing up. Our estrogen may be through the roof in terms of normal levels and may even reflect in our moods and menstrual cycles if we are female.

Prolactin can also be high raising concern for damage within the pituitary gland, which gives way for the very possibility of damage to the hypothalamus as well. No wonder our levels are all off. But, it does not end there. Our adrenal glands are now taxed as the brain is not communicating the correct response and hormones are flooding the system. Our not so little episodes of "fight-or flight" are having our cortisol levels increased by being pumped out increasingly and we end up being in disarray. Our calm peacefulness of homeostasis of a well-functioning body has been overtaken by disorder and confusion; and we really feel it as well as exhibit it. Unfortunately, many doctors are only trying to treat the symptoms and not the cause.

Our discomforts, stiffness and pain are met with a host of new medications being offered, that comes with an overwhelming amount of side-effects that only leave us wondering if we will ever be well again. Well, many of the drugs offered for auto-immune disorders suppress our already compromised immune system which leaves us vulnerable to any pathogen coming our way, and that would make us want to avoid life further. But, we do not really want to avoid life, we just want to avoid what causes the symptoms, and what causes the overwhelming stimuli. Sure, we would like to avoid pathogens, germs, viruses, bacteria, et cetera, but we don't want to avoid life because now we have to worry about our weakened immune system too.

When we have been diagnosed with an auto-immune disease or disorder, we learn that our body is attacking itself, thinking it is foreign. Our immune system is overactive, and it no longer recognizes our cells as being our own. As our own immune system attacks, more inflammation is caused which gives way to feelings of stiffness, swelling and pain in our joints. Our doctors may not even know exactly which auto-immune disorder we may have now developed as there are many with similar and overlapping symptoms. Our blood work will reveal a fluctuation in homeostasis as our levels will surely be altered, giving us some insight into what is going on within us physiologically.

We may have a positive ANA (antinuclear antibody), meaning autoantibodies are present, though does not necessarily mean there is a disease process started as some medications can cause a positive ANA as well as be present in an otherwise healthy individual. These antibodies are proteins made by the white blood cells and normally recognize and fight off germs in the body. They help the body do its job by fighting invaders and staying healthy. The antibody will recognize the "foreign" invaders and then recruit other proteins and cells to fight in the battle, which then causes inflammation. But, when they make a mistake between identifying normal healthy cells and proteins from the invaders, the antibodies become labeled as autoantibodies.

These autoantibodies cause the body to start attacking itself; friendly fire that's not so friendly. When these "antibodies" attack proteins within a cell's nucleus, they are then called antinuclear antibodies. If there is the presence of a large amount of these ANA's then that could very well indicate an auto-immune disease/disorder present within the body. Blood work testing for ANA could reveal the onset of various auto-immune diseases such as Rheumatoid Arthritis, Lupus, Mixed Connective Tissue Disease, Psoriatic Arthritis, Sjogren's Syndrome, Scleroderma, even Fibromyalgia, and many more.

Other lab work that will most likely be taken will be to check for Rheumatoid Factor—proteins that attack healthy tissue, anti-CCP (anti-cyclic citrullinated peptide)—presents early in a disease process of Rheumatoid Arthritis, ESR (erythrocyte sedimentation rate)—measuring degree of inflammation, and CRP (C-reactive protein)—a marker for inflammation, as well as other tests as per your doctor or Rheumatoid Specialist.

Though we may have a number of tests ordered, we may not end up with an answer. We may only hear the term "Mixed Connective Tissue Disease" by doctors as we present with symptoms similar to many auto-immune disorders including Lupus and Rheumatoid Arthritis; especially when we also present with Raynaud's Phenomenon, often exhibiting fingers and toes suddenly turning white and even bluish when exposed to colder temperatures, due to lack of blood circulation. Raynaud's is frequently experienced with Fibromyalgia as well.

We could oftentimes experience numbness and tingling as well—which all could lead to poor healing if our digits (fingers and toes) are injured. Mixed Connective Tissue Disease damages the muscle fibers, making them feel sore and weak and can be present in both the hips and shoulders. The lungs can also be affected as fluid builds up around the lungs causing shortness of breath which could lead to affecting the tissue around the air sacs (alveoli) of the lung, possibly causing pulmonary hypertension (high blood pressure in the lung's arteries) which is very serious and dangerous. This can all weaken the heart, occasionally leading to heart failure presenting symptoms of shortness of breath, fatigue, and fluid retention. Kidneys may also be involved, in up to 25% of cases, as is also fever, abdominal pain and swollen lymph nodes. Though this may sound very scary, and it is, it is not as detrimental as say Lupus actually is, because Lupus negatively affects multiple bodily systems with complications often accompanying. In severe cases of Rheumatoid Arthritis, organs and body systems may be affected as well as joints with worn cartilage and bone.

This is not meant to scare you, but rather to educate you to pay attention to your body and the symptoms it is giving you as they are clues to what is going on within. Additionally, doctors often refer to the term "Mixed Connective Tissue Disease" when they are unable to pin point exactly which auto-immune disease you may have. Because symptoms overlap, and blood work is not always conclusive, yet the patient still experiences very real symptoms that may change, wax and wane, and also experience new ones, it is sometimes a difficult puzzle to piece together.

Just do not ever give up or give in to discouragement as there is much help available to help you daily with your everyday needs. Just like when you had a brain injury, somehow help found you, unexpectedly. I remember my oldest son generously and faithfully drove me to my physical therapy appointments. That was such an appreciated and welcomed Blessing that made my day, each time. This is not a time for fear, but for courage at its grandest. This is a huge giant before you. With that being said, you do not have to backdown. You can stand up to it and fight back. You can get back up and keep going forward and hang onto hope; hope for a better day every time you fall, and hope for a better tomorrow with many good tomorrows. There are many natural ways to help so read on through and find both hope and joy in your heart.

Fear thou not; for I *am* with thee: be not dismayed; for I *am* thy God: I will strengthen thee; yea, I will help thee; yea, I will uphold thee with the right hand of my righteousness.
Isaiah 41:10 KJV

Have not I commanded thee? Be strong and of a good courage; be not afraid, neither be thou dismayed: for the LORD thy God *is* with thee whithersoever thou goest.
Joshua 1:9 KJV

O LORD my God, I cried unto thee, and thou
hast healed me.
Psalm 30:2 KJV

I WILL love thee, O LORD, my strength. The
LORD *is* my rock, and my fortress, and my
deliverer; my God, my strength, in whom I will
trust; my buckler, and the horn of my salvation,
and my high tower. I will call upon the LORD,
who is worthy to be praised: so shall I be
saved from mine enemies.
Psalm 18:1-3 KJV

So, What About Fibromyalgia?

In addition to the many auto-immune disorders that can be diagnosed, perhaps several within one person, as symptoms overlap causing confusion, two corresponding disorders and recently as well as frequently heard of lately are Chronic Fatigue Syndrome and its counterpart Fibromyalgia, though they technically are not considered or classified as auto-immune, even though Fibromyalgia was once believed to be arthritic in nature and an arthritis related condition. Laboratory tests often reveal that Fibromyalgia sufferers typically have low inflammatory markers, whereas with auto-immune disorders the inflammatory markers are much higher; because the body is attacking itself producing inflammation. The attention of Fibromyalgia is now directed to the nerves, brain and blood vessels with regard to communication, the Central Nervous System and blood flow.

Both Chronic Fatigue Syndrome and Fibromyalgia very often overlap in other disorders, concerning symptoms that are present in conjunction with an actual auto-immune disease such as Lupus, Rheumatoid Arthritis and many more. It is estimated that more than one quarter of the people diagnosed with an auto-immune disease also display Fibromyalgia and Chronic Fatigue. These two seem to go hand in hand and when they branch out into auto-immune disorders, such as Rheumatoid Arthritis with the similarity of symptoms, it can be very debilitating for anyone going through the experience of dealing with the symptoms of added pain and fatigue on a daily basis.

Fibromyalgia is estimated to affect 5 million adults in the United States alone. Both CFS (Chronic Fatigue Syndrome) and Fibromyalgia are characterized in people by extreme exhaustion, brain fog feeling and many times insomnia—despite being severely exhausted and wanting to just sleep. Sleep cycles are often broken, once finally falling asleep, with wakefulness throughout the night; often noticing Restless Leg Syndrome as well.

You may start to notice upon waking up to start your day, stiffness, joint pain and tender spots of pain in your feet as you start to walk. Moving around more seems to initially ease the pain, to only have it return once you slow down or get up from a sitting or lying position. In a way it makes you feel like you need to keep moving, through the pain, in order to feel better.

Other debilitating symptoms of Fibromyalgia include widespread musculoskeletal and nerve pain with amplified painful sensations, affecting the way the brain perceives pain. The brain mistakes normal touch sensations for painful ones and produces real painful sensation awareness in response. The signaled sensations can include tingling, burning, numbness and even sharp pains that can be so intense on the skin's surface, including the toes, that even the most, gentlest touch of a finger, feather or air, even light bedsheets on the bed for instance, can send a signal of sharp, excruciating needle-like and sharp "shards of glass"- like, sliver pain sensations, making it difficult to sleep, walk, or function normally. Taking a shower can become challenging as the water can intensify the "burning" sensation on a particular body part, as it splashes the body. When pain affects the feet or lower extremities, it can affect mobility. The intense sensations can last anywhere from a few brief moments to several hours and even days.

In addition to pain and touch sensitivity, Fibromyalgia symptoms can also include environmental sensitivity through smells, sounds and sights, migraines and chronic tension headaches, TMJ disorders (temporomandibular joint disorders), muscle and joint stiffness, muscle spasms, anxiety, depression, irritable bowel syndrome, short-term memory difficulties, problems with concentration and comprehension, brain fog, vision changes, fatigue with exhaustion, muscle twitching, trouble sleeping with frequent waking often due to restless leg syndrome, creepy crawly sensations on skin, Raynaud's Syndrome, and even endometriosis, all of which easily can lead to depression.

There are additional painful tender points at areas of: top of shoulders, back of head, between shoulder blades, front sides of neck, upper chest, elbows, upper hips, sides of hips and inner knees. Sometimes we may not realize having these tender points, until they're touched, and then, "Wow"! Something that can normally be a light touch can feel like a hard punch; I learned this as my husband playfully tapped my shoulder, which sent me off into a "Ouch, what was that?" response. I also can wake up with such pain that it seems to affect my entire limb as it actually feels limp and unmovable because of the pain.

There can however also be reduced sensations to stimuli compared to prior experiencing Fibromyalgia, as in the sensations of hands and feet as there may have been a time where you could not stand to have your feet tickled, but now, you could sit there and clearly take the touch sensation without moving or even twitching. Of course, these are the times when we are not experiencing a flare or increase in heightened sensations. This can also affect the hands as there seems to be more of a dullness or even a numbness sensation.

So, what is going on here? There may be an excessive amount of nerve fibers called arteriole-venule shunts. It is now thought that these fibers have a direct link to Fibromyalgia pain sensations. This can explain the extreme pain felt in hands, legs and feet at times due to the excess blood vessels in the hands, legs and feet. Though it was once thought that these nerve fibers only played a role in regulating blood flow at a subconscious level, it has now been proven that these blood vessel endings also play a role in our "conscious" sensations as well, for instance touch and the sensation of pain. This unregulated blood flow can cause extreme sharp pain, muscle cramping, achiness, and feelings of extreme fatigue. It is, in a sense, our pain sensors are not working properly, and our stiffness and achy joints make it difficult to even get our knickers on in a hurry, especially if someone is about to walk into the room we're in. We may fumble in angst and haste thinking, "Hello, Houston—we have a big problem! A little help here, please!"

So, as we go about our day full of fatigue and pain, for myself, I can almost hear Scotty saying in response to Captain Kirk, as Kirk asks him to divert more power saying, "Full power to the shields, Mister Scott" (the infamous line in Star Trek), "Given them all we got!" to captain. I yearn to offer my own response, "But, I need more! Send in the turbo boosters, or whatever you've got!" As I sigh in desperation I announce, "I'm under attack! Red Alert! Photon torpedoes! Anything?" Boy, doesn't it feel like that? After all, we need more energy, not to mention protection from the invading symptoms wrecking our days! So, shields up! I can relate to the character "Bones" McCoy, in fact I love his humor and personality, when his hands are tied in not being able to "fix this", when something is a matter of physics and not medicine; because he's a doctor, not a physicist. I don't know about you, but I'm not a doctor, nor a physicist. I am a person most likely just like you, going through the journey of life with life events and physical ailments happening. So, I am determined to find the joy throughout this, or any other life-altering challenge. How about you? After all, we should all want to "live long and prosper"!

Perhaps, I should watch an old Star Trek episode or movie to get my mind off the pain. Distraction, when it's a good kind, can and does help in many ways. Whatever your fancy, as long as it is safe and does not hurt anybody. We could read, meditate, pray, try to learn something new, exercise, play a game, listen to relaxing music that brings back good memories, share meaningful company and conversation with someone, and even watch or engage in something joyful or funny that brings a smile and laughter to our immediate world. You know what they say, "laughter is good medicine"; and it sure is!

Because this can be so debilitating, painful and exhausting, depression is easily brought on; because the ongoing symptoms are depressing to go through. When we don't get enough sleep, due to restless legs, being that we're still moving trying to get comfortable from leg discomfort and creepy crawly sensations, it only adds to our exhaustion. Potassium rich foods such as avocados and bananas may be of help for restless legs and leg discomfort as they help with proper nerve function. Ashwagandha is also beneficial in supporting sleep and rejuvenates the body from stress related exhaustion, helping to avoid depression-like symptoms. Doctors generally prescribe narcotic pain relief along with anti-depressants and anti-convulsant drugs; but the risks of taking those can bring about a whole new source of problems and side-effects which can present your body with additional risks and complications. When this is presented to you, do your research reading through all side-effects and drug interactions. If you can, go the natural route first.

- **St. John's Wort**—an herbal OTC (over the counter) remedy can be effective in treating mild depression with much less unwanted side-effects but is not as effective in treating major depression. St. John's Wort may increase sensitivity to the sun as it is photosensitive and may also reduce effectiveness of birth control pills. Talking with your healthcare provider or naturopath along with research will help you to make an informed decision.

- **SAMe**—can help impaired brain and bodily functions, as it benefits both brain, and joint activity, and can be a treatment for depression, arthritis, as well as a liver tonic. **However--SAMe should not be used for depression with bipolar disorders unless under medical supervision due to the possibility of worsening bipolar episodes.

  Cymbalta however, which is often prescribed for fibromyalgia symptoms, including depression, peripheral neuropathy, back pain and also arthritic pain, carries many risks including hallucinations, nausea, vomiting and diarrhea, bloody stools, seizures, abdominal pain, increase in blood pressure as well as low pressure resulting in loss of consciousness, dizziness, lightheadedness, decrease in libido, twitching, unexplained fever, blisters, rash, trouble breathing, liver toxicity, and increase in suicidal tendencies—to name a few! WOW! Makes you wonder, just because those nice commercials with people, families and friends, having fun enjoying themselves, and are set to soft music while all the nasty side-effects are either written or spoken softly in the background, does not mean that this is a safe medication or the only choice for your symptoms. This is deception at its finest! Don't' let the imagery or nice melody distract you from the facts. Your health is what matters, not the drug companies pocketbook!

Gabapentin (Neurontin) is another widely prescribed medication that is not only used for seizures (as it was approved as an anti-convulsant, not for pain), but is also now frequently being prescribed for neuropathic pain, hot flashes, Restless Leg Syndrome, insomnia, post-operative pain, brain injury patients, many auto-immune disorders, as well as Fibromyalgia, and even anxiety, mostly due to the opioid epidemic; but it is literally killing people.

In light of this epidemic, Gabapentin is considered to be an alternative to opioid use in treating pain, however, the side-effects are far too many including being linked to numerous deaths and also an increase in several emergency room visits upon taking the drug.

Some minor side-effects, if they are even considered minor, include dizziness, double vision, swelling of hands, ankles and feet, pain, seizures, bipolar disorders, allergic reactions, rash, trouble breathing, swollen lymph nodes, severe dizziness, loopy zombie-like feelings, depression and suicide. Now, those are not minor in any way and cause exactly what you are trying to prevent! Note: Monitor carefully when stopping Gabapentin as it could cause seizures!

***The big problem with Gabapentin is that it is known to suppress breathing, causing respiratory depression and death, as are opioids. When opioids are also taken, as they are absurdly often prescribed together for severe pain, the absorption of Gabapentin within the body is also increased, further increasing risk. Not only so, but if it is taken within 120 day's-time, a risk is still there as some opioids are long-acting. This is a huge drug to drug interaction that needs to be addressed before more people die!

*** Do most of us, or any of us know the risks before taking Gabapentin? I would say not because numbers don't lie. When we are in pain, we become desperate and look for relief any way we can. We go to the doctors, trusting they have our best interests in mind, but when this drug is being prescribed like candy without telling patients of its high risks, and not making sure there is not, has not been, or will not be any opioid use in conjunction with or within 120 days, there is potentially a grave mistake.

Another thing to note is the effectiveness of Gabapentin for pain relief. For most people in various studies ranging over 16 plus years, the results are that it works no better than, and even less than, an over-the-counter NSAID (non-steroidal anti-inflammatory drug). So, why is this drug being prescribed for so many things, other than what it was approved for?

Additionally, to add to this CNS depressant are the risks of also taking benzodiazepines (other CNS depressants) for anxiety, panic disorders, insomnia and Restless Leg Syndrome, which can further compromise our health and life. We all need to become accountable and knowledgeable to what we are taking into our bodies. All doctors involved in a patient's care need to know and recognize the risks of what their patients are being prescribed and/or taking from all sources including any street drugs as well as what is prescribed from any specialist, such as Rheumatology, Neurology, pain management doctors, and also primary care physicians; as do pharmacists as well before filling a prescription. It is equally important that the patient be honest as their life can depend upon it; in avoiding a deadly drug interaction.

When a doctor prescribes something, ask questions. Ask why, for how long, side-effects, minimal dose, alternatives, et cetera. They may not however always tell you the truth. I was once prescribed a potent and pretty lethal anti-seizure medication, by a neurologist, when I was diagnosed with a Traumatic Brain Injury and Post-Concussion Syndrome. This person's "reasoning" was that though I had a TBI, PCS doesn't exist past two weeks, therefore he thought it was in my head along with my "menopausal age"—I was 46 at the time. I wanted to say, "Hey Doc, so, if you get a blow to the head and end up with a Traumatic Brain Injury with ongoing concussion-like symptoms, it must mean that you are menopausal—though you are male. Oh yeah, it's also in your head!" That was the stupidest comment I ever heard a doctor say to me, especially because I am female. To think, he gets paid well for this lack of care!

So, even though, there may be a big-name doctor in a thriving practice, (how and why, I will never fully understand), we must educate ourselves on everything we put into our bodies—including and especially medications. The last line of defense stops with you! The doctor may prescribe a medication, a drug, and the pharmacist may fill the prescription, but, it is you who are taking it, putting it into your mouth and swallowing it at the risk of your health, potentially having grave effects.

As far as anti-seizure drugs, like that one above is concerned, read all the potential side-effects as the risks may out-way any benefit. You do not want to die taking a medication! The whole point of going to the doctor in the first place is to get better, not worse! You really must come to an informed decision when it comes to your health; we all must! Our very lives, our futures and our quality of life depends on it.

'How did I get this Fibromyalgia in the first place?', one may be wondering. Especially since Fibromyalgia has gotten a bad rap from many main-stream doctors as being a "made-up" disease—that is until they've either experienced it or someone close to them has, (much like any other "hidden" condition or injury, including a brain injury), because it may be difficult to pinpoint and therefore, even harder to understand. Since it is so inter-related, having overlapping symptoms to many auto-immune diseases, it can be confusing, especially if we've heard or are faced with any skepticism regarding the condition. Oftentimes, unfortunately, doctors will dismiss Fibromyalgia as being either psychological or even psychiatric in nature, though it is a very real condition involving the nervous system and brain, triggered by an event such as an injury, especially a brain injury, and even by a surgical procedure, infection, or anything that can damage the brain by causing an interruption or even lack of oxygen.

TBI & Fibromyalgia

Although Fibromyalgia can sometimes run in families, as there may be certain genetic mutations making susceptibility more probable, along with some illnesses or infections that may also act as a trigger to bring about the condition and even aggravate an existing one, more oftentimes it is not the cause. Studies have been conducted that ask patients coming in with symptoms of Fibromyalgia, if they have ever had a brain injury. The answers were outstanding with overwhelming numbers of "yes's"!

Now, many times we don't even realize that we have had a brain injury, that is unless it was so detrimental and impactful that we could not function as normal. Many times, our bumps to the head, our quick jolts, (even from some amusement park rides) are enough to cause damage on the inside, though we may mistakenly just take it as minor, like having our clock, or bell rung. However, there is no such thing as minor because concussions can cause lasting damage no matter how minor, no matter if our pupils dilate and react to light or not. Concussions are trauma caused to the brain, period; and our brain is the control center of everything else!

We may try to accept the stance that "it's only a small hit", or "it's okay", or even "I'll be fine, I can take it", but it will catch up to you and the more times it happens, the more your body goes through a huge inflammatory process, which ultimately changes everything. Effects may take time, they may take months, years even, but when you receive that sudden news of an auto-immune disease popping up or the often, unexplained Fibromyalgia, think back to an injury to your brain, and let your doctor know.

For the sake of this book and the very likelihood and probability of trauma being a significant and root cause of Fibromyalgia, both physical as well as emotional trauma, it is a contributing factor; the key trigger point. Post-Traumatic Stress as well as Traumatic Brain Injury cause a great deal of stress and inflammation within the body, miscommunication of hormones and rewiring of circuitry within the Central Nervous System. With this being said, Post-Traumatic Stress has also indeed been linked to Fibromyalgia, as has TBI.

Since the brain is the master computer system for the entire body, when signals are sent to the brain via the body in a brain injured individual, they are all garbled, distorted and scrambled making it difficult to decipher. The highway of information signals that travel through the spinal cord are not always getting through correctly when there is damage to neurons, and/or nerves themselves. Communication is either down or altered. Since the brain controls the pain centers, therefore the perception of pain and any sensations can be greatly altered. It does not matter how big of a head injury that occurred as even the seemingly slightest one can cause a host of problems.

Inside the brain are bony structures protruding outward, with the brain being soft and delicate. When a bump to the head, a quick jolt, or a fast shaking motion happens, the brain bounces all over the place within the skull, much like gelatin bounces when shaken. The brain bounces off the inside walls of the skull receiving contusions (bruising) within the brain as well as stretching, tearing and severed axons resulting in loss and even death of neurons, making the synapses, the connections within the brain, severely compromised.

The resultant effects, depending upon the lobes damaged amount to a host of immediate symptoms affecting learning, comprehension, memory, speech, walking, pain, balance and proprioception issues, vision disturbances, light and sound sensitivity, emotional and personality changes, sleep disturbances, hormonal imbalances, concentration problems, fatigue and a host of other symptoms. A brain injury should never, ever be taken lightly, but watched, even over the course of years for any development of auto-immune disorders or Fibromyalgia symptoms. A brain injury could very well be the catalyst to your next adventure in life, as it may have only just begun.

When we start to notice a lengthy fatigue, chronic if you will, that may be a clue something is going on, and it's not just your age. Don't buy into people's opinions of "age related" symptoms telling you, "Well, you are getting older." Ah, that's not it! I remember explaining my symptoms to a "family member" only to have them respond in kind to the "age" excuse. "Yeah, I'm not that old!" is always my response! As they typically live the sedentary lifestyle where you could out-run them any day—if only you didn't have this darn fatigue. Grrrrr. Anyway, we are better and stronger for going through this because we are only given what we truly can handle. So, guess we can handle this, and perhaps, they cannot.

But, this fatigue, does kick my butt! I have found that Ganoderma and Schisandra Berry help tremendously. I talk more about them both in the diet section. When Chronic Fatigue Syndrome (CFS) comes on gradually over a period of time, it is most often triggered by a hormonal imbalance—enter in hormonal imbalance resulting from damage to the hypothalamus in the brain via a brain injury for the sake of this book.

CFS can also occur with a Candida overgrowth (brain gut connection) and can accompany an auto-immune disorder—brought on by a disruption in homeostasis, caused by inflammation due to diet, toxins—chemicals/insecticides, mold, fungus, parasites, infections, environment, and injury (such as in the case of a brain injury) that causes great inflammation that has a butterfly effect throughout the entire body.

When a Candida (fungal infection) overgrowth happens, there can be certain symptoms experienced that overlap with other ailments. These include: a weakened immune system, UTI (urinary tract infection), joint pain, hormonal imbalance, low sex drive, chronic sinus issues and allergies, digestive problems, brain fog, exhaustion, bad breath, cravings for sweets, and a white coating on the tongue, (Thrush). There are different species of Candida, one being a yeast infection affecting the mouth, intestinal tract and vagina known as Candida Albicans, and another more serious known as Candida Auris that has been named a "superbug" making it a dangerous health threat as it spreads through Candida biofilms, adhering to surfaces such as bedrails, catheters and more, that is multiple drug resistant.

Normally Candida Albicans (yeast infection) is not serious, unless of course an immune system is already compromised, weakened and not functioning properly because then it can travel to other area of the body including the bloodstream and also membranes around both the heart and brain.

Candida is a fungus that when it is within normal levels in the body, helps aid in digestion and nutrient absorption, but when it is overproduced, that is when the symptoms begin, breaking down the walls within the intestinal lining, penetrating the blood stream, and releasing biproduct toxins causing "leaky gut syndrome". This all disrupts the body's natural pH balance leading to an out of control Candida over growth which create a systemic problem for the entire body with many symptoms arising. In order to properly fight this overgrowth infection, a properly functioning immune system is required along with good "gut" bacteria. You may find that you have even developed new "allergies", sensitivities and intolerances to foods such as eggs, dairy, corn and of course gluten containing foods. They may affect you like never before, sending you off into a symptomatic filled world. When this happens, our immune system must be fixed.

Candida can additionally be caused by stress, and an injury such as a brain injury causes a great deal of stress on the body which leads to inflammation and an overgrowth of yeast. Also, Candida can be caused by the use of antibiotics as they also kill our "good" gut bacteria, birth control pills when consumed with refined sugar, cancer treatments, and even oral corticosteroids—inhalants for asthma (don't stop your inhaler) just swish or clean your mouth out after use to avoid Candida of the mouth. If mouth Candida (Thrush) is suspected, swish additionally with coconut oil and a drop of essential clove oil.

Since Candida thrives on sugar, much like cancer growth does, people suffering from Diabetes are at high risk as there are higher glucose levels often present. Monitor for any developing symptoms of Candida.

Again, since this Candida involves the immune system as it grows rapidly with a weakened, compromised, underdeveloped or unregulated immune system, it is surely a great concern not only for small children, infants, and the elderly, but also for people dealing with inflammatory disorders and auto-immune diseases. Since the immune system is not working properly, we are at risk and should monitor for signs and symptoms of Candida overgrowth such as Thrush, yeast and urinary tract infections, sinus infections, mood changes of anxiety, depression, irritability, panic attacks, hormonal imbalances, intestinal issues, brain fog, skin and nail fungus-- including Athlete's foot, and chronic fatigue.

If Candida is suspected, you may need to go for blood work, a urinalysis and possibly a stool sample, depending on your healthcare provider's recommendation. Treatment for Candida overgrowth is the process of ridding the body of excess Candida through the digestive tract along with the bringing in of warrior fighters to help in this battle—like fermented foods such as Kefir, Kombucha, also probiotic yogurts and vegetables. You can even add cinnamon to yogurt for a double punch knock-out for that Candida "bad guy", as cinnamon is also anti-fungal, antibacterial and anti-parasitic. The idea is to cleanse out the bad, to detox, and bring in the good. You will need to heal your gut, so your gut and brain connection can do their best at running your body, keeping you healthy and disease free.

There are many helpful natural ways to treat Candida. You can purchase a natural Candida cleanse to rid your body of the fungus. You may also want to add foods to your diet such as garlic, having 2-4 crushed cloves a day during treatment and also keeping garlic (a lesser amount) in your regular diet. Garlic is naturally anti-fungal due to its sulfur containing compounds making it a natural fungus fighter. You can also directly apply garlic to an affected area; but it does stink. Hey, at least you won't have to worry about getting bit by a vampire.

Coconut oil is another perfect anti-fungal necessity to one's diet as it truly does have so many benefits, both internally and topically, plus it smells much better than garlic; but still try the garlic internally. I discuss some benefits of coconut oil in the diet section coming up. Coconut oil can be applied directly, 3-4 times per day, to a fungal infection as it can to any skin irritation or even dryness. You will not need much as it melts on your skin's surface and covers the area well in a smooth glide. Coconut oil really is a must to add to your diet and helps heal and also maintain gut health. You may want to add 1-3 Tbs. of coconut oil daily for best health results and benefits.

Additionally, tea tree oil, oil of oregano and olive oil have also been useful in treating Candida as is cranberry juice. Yes, your mom and perhaps your grandma was right when they said, "Drink your cranberry juice"; but it must be whole cranberry juice, not cocktail—cocktail means sugar and that will just feed your overgrowth of Candida even more.

A liquid vegetable broth is a great way to jump start your cleanse of letting go of the toxins hanging around inside. You can use vegetables such as garlic, celery, kale, onions, throw in olive leaves—all organic is best, along with mineral dense sea salt or Himalayan salt and water, and "bam"—goodbye Candida. Boil, discard vegetables and sip throughout the day. Bone broths are also a perfect way to heal your gut and is discussed further in the diet section, but for Candida overgrowth, try this vegetable remedy. Isn't it just so amazing what we have naturally growing in creation, foods that are not only nutritious and good for us, but also healing. I just have to say, "Wow!"

You will also want to eliminate sugars from your diet along with grains, fruit, alcohol and starches for about five days of cleansing—sugar would be wise to eliminate indefinitely and completely, or at least only use sparingly as it is detrimental to your health. Try eating organically steamed vegetables but avoiding starchy ones such as potatoes, carrots, beets, (those root vegetables) just during a detox; afterward is fine. Make sure to drink plenty of water continually, just like when you initially had the brain injury and realized the brain is comprised of so much water and requires it for healthy cognitive function. With Candida removal, drink even more. Yes, more!

Remember in my previous books I had mentioned the importance of making your body more alkaline to help remain disease free, well that goes for this as well. If you do not remember, or have not read it, know this, that acidity produces disease in the body and the sugar feeds it. A great way, every day, is to take apple cider vinegar with the mother; that is the full chain of amino acids. You can add it to a glass of water to protect your teeth's enamel and throw in some ginger for many health benefits including for pain and inflammation, and also add cinnamon, fresh lemon juice (anti-fungal, alkalizes and detoxes), and turmeric for pain and inflammation control (with crushed black pepper for increased absorption). Normally I would add natural honey but for a Candida overgrowth, I would not. We want to rid the body of Candida and not have any fruits or sugar for these few days at least, even natural sugar (honey). You can also add apple cider vinegar to your bath, and just go and relax, listen to music, grab a book—maybe this one.

The possibility of having an overgrowth of Candida should be discussed with your healthcare provider. Don't worry or be concerned by being embarrassed as there are so many causes; that is why it is so common but needs to be treated nonetheless. The sooner you treat this and get rid of the overgrowth taking over your body, the better you will feel.

With CFS you may experience bowel disturbances or disorders, increased thirst, weight gain, recurring sinus and respiratory infections and low libido, to name a few. Fibromyalgia sufferers can experience this along with severe pain either localized or all over the body which is sensitive to touch, caused by shortening or tightening of muscles due to decreased bodily energy. This "chronic" muscle pain then triggers nerve pain and the overall sensitization, which then gives a feeling of brain pain. But, if energy production can be restored, it will help the muscles to relax, therefore reduce the pain. Additionally, nerve pain, neuropathy, or neuropathic pain that so often accompanies Fibromyalgia can be helped by adding Evening Primrose Oil to your supplementation regimen as it has shown to improve overall nerve function. Topical Lidocaine is sometimes prescribed to offer additional anesthetic effects.

Since neurons in the hypothalamus control functions such as sleep, temperature, blood flow, blood pressure, and hormones, it often decreases its function in order to protect the individual in the face of an overwhelming stress; with CFS and Fibromyalgia being the circuit breaker or a blown fuse. When we can't sleep deeply enough, the time when the body heals and restores itself, our immune system then stops working effectively resulting in increased pain with lack of energy needed for our muscles, along with muscle shortening. This results in an energy crisis throughout our entire body and an increase in fatigue. Yeah, we know that feeling, for sure.

The hypothalamic suppression and resulting disconnect throughout the body to function properly brings about a host of unwelcomed feelings and symptoms that most often doctors struggle to effectively realize and diagnose.   Since proper hypothalamic function is absolutely critical to falling asleep and staying asleep, we may start to notice a problem as we struggle to get a good 7-8 hours of restful sound sleep in per night.   Melatonin (a hormone produced by the pineal gland that regulates sleep), 5-HTP (amino acid precursor to serotonin, created by L-tryptophan aids serotonin and melatonin to help with sleep/wake cycles) and passionflower (a wild flower that promotes better sleep by reducing insomnia, anxiety, and inflammation), are all helpful in combatting lack of and trouble with sleep; as is healthy levels of serotonin to help balance mood and restful sleep.

Additionally, since the hypothalamus is at the heart of the control center for the body, and the communication source to the adrenal glands for producing the correct amounts of hormones, periodically having a hormonal blood work panel drawn is essential. Upon evaluation you may want to consider adding Ashwagandha and Schisandra Berry to your vitamin and supplement routine to help aid in supporting proper adrenal function, along with possibly taking a "low dose" DHEA (dehydroepiandrosterone—a hormone made in the adrenal glands) under your health care provider's supervision, as many over the counter doses are way too high, to properly balance things out and help with adrenal insufficiency; at the very least, ask a pharmacist for recommended dosage.

Helping to restore the body will encompass diet as well as exercise. Our diets must not consist of coming out of a box, nor through the dollar menu at our local fast food restaurant. Think of it this way, if a meal is only about a buck, prepared, after the cost of the "food product", employees, and business/building expenses, you have to wonder, what the initial cost of that product really is—therefore the quality, or lack thereof. Fresh whole foods are best and minimal cooking to enhance nutrition, vitamin and mineral content. We are going to need our vitamins especially B-12 (separately, if supplementing because too much "B-6" in B-Complex can cause nerve damage), C and D, antioxidants, minerals—especially zinc, magnesium and selenium, amino acids, and natural foods and herbs to restore our body's health at an optimal level. Additionally, capsaicin, the active compound in cayenne pepper, is useful in helping treat peripheral neuropathy that so often accompanies Fibromyalgia. Just think, food is our medicine. We will discuss more on food later.

Other helpful tips in managing auto-immune disorders or Fibromyalgia are to include accepting support and help from others when you need it, additional rest times, sufficient sleep, avoiding stress (we don't want to add any more), pace ourselves so we minimize getting over-whelmed and take frequent break times, exercise regularly (walking is perfect as it is aerobic in nature and very helpful with joint mobility), deep breathing and relaxation exercises with slow movements, and also massage therapy can even help—if you can even be touched that is. Wait for a good time that you are able as it will benefit the muscles and soft tissues, improve range of motion and increase the body's natural production of pain killers as it relieves stress and anxiety.

Despite what any of the blood tests taken may reveal, or the many symptoms we may be experiencing, the diagnose we have been given—or not, as our doctor may not quite know yet, we must not give into discouragement nor be dismayed. Think of this period, this moment in time, as yet another life changing event in our journey of life, with an opportunity to change our lifestyle and diet for the better; your lifestyle and diet for a better and much healthier you. This can be an opportunity for growth despite what it may seem like. This very well can be the catalyst for positive change that will overflow into family and perhaps even friends.

Think of this as a time in your life to start getting your priorities straight, that is your health and well-being, which encompasses all aspects including physical, emotional, spiritual, financial and relational. If you think about it, what good is your finances if you are really sick, debilitated and can't enjoy a real quality of life? How are your relationships now going to be affected as a direct result of your new diagnosis, both relational as well as professional? If you can't physically move about comfortably due to pain and stiffness, is it affecting your emotional state in how you now feel about yourself as well as your life?

With those questions to ponder on, you can't let this or anything else defeat you! No! You, we all, really must endure what we are going through to the best of our ability, the best way we can and with as much joy as we can. We really must keep moving forward, in a forward motion, rather than becoming stagnant or frozen within our circumstance or even falling into a trap to regress backwards. We cannot live in the past with any regrets and we can't be stuck there with all the "what if's". We all must persevere with hope for our future. To do that we must have courage to try, to keep trying and to never give up!

This new diagnosis may just be the catalyst for a positive change. You can do it and there are plenty of natural ways to help you. The medical field is used to treating the symptoms and not the root cause of them. Thankfully there are practitioners called naturopaths who are trained naturopathic physicians who are very knowledgeable and skilled on the human body in terms of how it functions as well as how it heals and what helps aid in the healing process. Therefore, they are also very knowledgeable on the best ways to treat as well as get to the underlying cause of symptoms through a holistic approach which is best for your body and overall health without disrupting it further; unlike traditional medicine which has its answers in the form of pharmaceutical drugs that mostly presents the body with further ill effects as it mostly masks symptoms.

Naturopaths focus on a proactive approach to prevention and healing, comprehensive diagnose and holistic treatment minimizing risks of harm to the body in any way as they help the body facilitate its own inherent ability to restore and maintain optimal health. A naturopathic physician will identify as well as remove the barriers or obstacles that are preventing good health by creating a healing environment both internally as well as externally.

Naturopaths treat a wide array of medical conditions and ailments and are equipped to treat any individual as well as an entire family. Some of the common ailments a naturopathic physician may treat are allergies, digestive issues, respiratory conditions, heart disease, fertility, obesity, cancer, menopause, hormonal imbalances, chronic fatigue, chronic pain, fibromyalgia, and auto-immune disorders. If you are diagnosed with any of these, and most likely you are or will be as a result of a disconnect in your body brought about by the huge inflammatory process of a brain injury, and further worsened by diet, then I urge you to seek out a naturopathic physician trained in holistic treatment through diet and nutrition, homeopathy, botanical medicine, hydrotherapy, mental health and well-being, and also naturopathic physical manipulation to aid in your care of a better healthier life. Get your life back and live the best you can.

Some naturopaths are also trained chiropractors which is a plus in dealing with the nervous system and all the disconnects going on within the body, as they are trained to realign the body and release any compression of the nerves that run along the entire spinal column up to the brain that could be blocking signals from the sensory neurons.

This can be an added benefit for headaches sufferers, due to lingering post-concussion symptoms as well as anyone dealing with auto-immune disorders and the many aches, pains and stiffness that also accompany it. Instant relief can be obtained as well as increased comfort and mobility through these highly trained and knowledgeable practitioners through chiropractor care and naturopathic healing as they get to the root causes of imbalances and disturbances within the human body and bring them back into alignment and homeostasis; complete well-being. Through a holistic healing approach, symptoms of imbalance, pain in the joints, muscles, tendons, ligaments, bones, and head can be relieved, and healing can start; all achieved through functional natural healing.

Now, most if not all, insurance companies will not cover these treatments, especially depending where you live, but can you really put a price on healing? If you think about it, you pay into your insurance company a pretty hefty amount and then most likely will still need to pay a co-pay on top of that, only to walk away with a prescription of a medication that has way too many side-effects that not only keep you sick, but many times destroys your immune system further (auto-immune sufferers, you know what I am talking about). You walk away frustrated and uncertain about your future, mistakenly thinking that this is it as you become discouraged beyond means. Your doctor may not even really know how to help you other than through drugs because they have an allegiance with the pharmaceutical industry, receiving as many "kickbacks" as their practice will allow, at the cost of patient's well-being. Ask yourself, "What is affected now?" Your physical health, emotional and mental health, your finances, your relationships and your hope for a positive change could all be affected from not receiving proper care.

However, there is hope because just one thought about a holistic approach may brighten your outlook. Just one visit can alter your perception of what really helps, as the amount of time they will spend with you, listening to you, examining you and every aspect of your environment that could be hurting your health. They can also help by identifying the causes of your ills, your pains and what is making your inflammation worse, in addition to treating you through natural means. Finally, you can have some answers that you have so longed for. Your body is crying out to you saying, "Help me, help you!" So, do what is helpful not harmful, so your body can get back to taking care of you.

You may need more than one visit, but at least take that first step to recovery and healing. Take that first step of hope, that leap of faith. What good is it to throw your money, your time and your sanity away to the medical industry that has become big business and you're still not getting any better, and maybe even possibly worse? Don't get me wrong, medicine and traditional medical doctors do have their place as well as medicine itself. The trouble lies when morals and integrity are replaced with greed to the patient's expense and the patients lose. There is a time and place for almost everything, but every ailment does not necessarily need a drug. So, don't give up! Have hope, there is help.

For those moments when we feel the "creepy crawly" sensations, ready to freak out because we think something may be crawling on us, yelling, "Get it off! Get it off!", only to find out it is our own hair, clothing, jewelry, or just a "nerve" sensation, we can just think of green pastures with no bugs. In my world that I often imagine, there are no bugs—except butterflies and ladybugs; bees maybe, for honey, because real natural honey is good. But the bugs don't come near me.

Since our Creator has made everything in our world, including all the natural healing plants, let's try some of them and experience the goodness, the healing properties all around us, in this big beautiful place we live, called earth. The beauty, the healing, is just surrounding us. We really do have all that we need because God supplies all of our need, according to His riches in Glory through Christ Jesus.

May the God of hope fill you with all joy and peace as you trust in him, so that you may overflow with hope by the power of the Holy Spirit.
Romans 15:13 NIV

But those who trust in the LORD will find new strength. They will soar high on wings like eagles. They will run and not grow weary. They will walk and not faint.
Isaiah 40:31 NLT

But Jesus beheld *them*, and said unto them, With men this is impossible; but with God all things are possible.
Matthew 19:26 KJV

THE LORD *is* my shepherd; I shall not want. He maketh me to lie down in green pastures: he leadeth me beside the still waters. He restoreth my soul: he leadeth me in the paths of righteousness for his name's sake. Yea, though I walk through the valley of the shadow of death, I will fear no evil: for thou *art* with me; thy rod and thy staff they comfort me. Thou preparest a table before me in the presence of mine enemies: thou anointest my head with oil; my cup runneth over. Surely goodness and mercy shall follow me all the days of my life: and I will dwell in the house of the LORD for ever.
Psalm 23:1-6 KJV

When Your World Comes Crashing Down

Those of us who have already suffered a brain injury and all that it entails, much of what I talk about in my previous two brain books, have already endured so much. We have come a long, long way and we have learned some things along that journey; enough to overflow and perhaps help others going through the same thing. We all know that having a brain injury is hard enough. Having it linger, the symptoms, for a very prolonged amount of time, as in living with Post-Concussion Syndrome, is truly life-altering and frustrating. Having another condition or disorder bloom out of the chaos of it all can be disheartening, super challenging and almost devastating. We may begin to feel helpless as well as hopeless even if we are starting to do the right things, eat the right foods, partake in the right beneficial therapies and see the right doctors compassionate enough and willing to get to the bottom of the root causes of our issues. Finding hope, can be the difference between joy and despair. But how, when all we're starting to feel is depressed?

Many times, a loss of hope derives from fear and lack of trust. We may feel lost in the midst of our circumstance and not really know where to turn next. We've been to doctors with anticipation in our hearts that we may finally have some answers, only to be crushed in spirit as their only solutions involved drugs to cover and mask our symptoms, though the problem still lies awake beneath the surface. We may have left physician office after physician office only to be disappointed, with much of the same resulting outcome along with a diagnosis of "anxiety", only to find that we are stuck in a valley of darkness, trapped in chains of the same diagnosis that does not really fit.

Painstakingly we pick other people's brain in a desperate search of the right doctor, one who will go the extra mile and is not concerned with the pharmaceutical industry's attempt to buy him or her, at the cost of their patients. Finally, we may find a good conscientious doctor, but guess what? They don't take our insurance. Grrrr! Now what? Our last glimmers of hope are fleeting fast. We may feel like our hands are tied, like were stuck in chains.

Some of us may give in to the victim sensation and wrongfully think that this is it. There's nothing that can be done except to take that pill and be labeled. However, we must not think like that. It is not over! We are still alive, here, breathing. If you are reading this, you know what? You are still here, given that gift of another day. You are breathing, and you can find joy even in these circumstances. There is always hope despite how we are feeling or what someone may say to us that brings us down. There is still hope.

We may very well feel weak, tired, in pain and greatly fatigued, but we are not alone. First of all, there are many others suffering the same and even worse than we are, and some of them have joy in their hearts along with hope for their futures. Wouldn't you like some of that, what they have, instead of despair and doubt? Though our worlds may be crashing down around us, we do not have to fall with it. We can rise above it! Not only are we not alone because others are experiencing difficult trials too and there is nothing new to our experiences that someone else has not or is not also familiar with, but we also have a friend that is closer than a brother and Who has experienced everything and more than we could ever imagine.

You may be either comforted right about now or jumpy and antsy in your seat for thinking upon this and wondering what is coming next. Though this truth may cause uneasiness in an unbeliever, it brings great comfort and peace, joy even, for a believer; a believer in Christ. Now I know perhaps your wall is going up at this moment but hear me out. I have a question for you to ponder on. Do you really want to go through this difficult situation and life-altering event alone with perhaps feelings of doubt, worry, anxiety, loneliness, loss of hope and despair? Or, would you like to be comforted, at peace with circumstances, have help and strength to get through, along with experience joy and also have lasting hope? Doesn't the second question sound much better, honestly? Be honest with yourself.

Now, you have to be true to yourself, because who else will. Maybe go to a quiet spot and ponder this. The choice is yours fully. The question is, "believe or not to believe?"; that truly is the question. That sums it up. Shakespeare had it right. Do we then have the will to want to be joy filled and free from the burdens that life throws us, the consequences of choices as well as the fall-out of injuries along with the various pains we feel, whether from physical, emotional, relational, financial, et cetera, brought our way? Do we long for comfort, freedom and forgiveness? Do we believe we, us ourselves, can actually have that? Can we believe that we can walk in our life with such a faith as well as grace, and a strength that is supernatural, not of our own? Well, we can, if we only believe. It comes down to "choice" in what or Who we believe in. When we choose to believe, it is undeniable as we begin to see God working in our own lives.

I am a faith filled person who does believe in God. I believe in Jesus Christ as my Savior and also my deliverer and healer out of the "pains" of my brain injury and now my auto-immune disorder and Fibromyalgia. After all, He is the Great Physician. Personally, He has showed up for me big time—I can no longer deny. He absorbs my pain, my anxiousness and my doubts and fills me with peace, comfort and joy in their stead. He brings me the help I need and gives me the strength I cannot come up with on my own to endure. He removes my worry and I am able to trust in Him and have real lasting hope, daily.

This is the only way I got through as far as I did and still am. He is my deliverer out of this and more. He is my fortress to hide in and my immovable rock. He is my anchor to be able to still hold on. He is my ultimate healer. Through faith in Christ is the only way; not in others or even myself. The world, family, friends, doctors and even including our own selves will inevitably let us down at some point. It can be extremely overwhelming. We will feel like we just "can't", anymore. But, you know what? Maybe, we can't, but God can! God can help us, and He will help us, if we will only let Him. I let Him. Will you let Him? This is far too hard to handle on our own.

He will move mountains for us and get us the help we so desperately need; through others, through nutrition, through helpful tools, through many means and ways. He will orchestrate events and bring to pass, outcomes that we need and even desire within our hearts. God is all-powerful, "Omnipotent" and nothing is too hard for Him, including our brain injuries or our auto-immune disorders, or even painful Fibromyalgia. He understands with compassion and is with us always and everywhere because He is "Omnipresent", everywhere at the same time. Since God is also "Omniscient", all-knowing, He knows exactly what we need when we truly need it. For all this, we can take comfort and just rest in Him.

We can look to Him and trust in Him for caring for us, for all our needs, and to strengthen us all the way through. Then we can experience peace and joy, when most others would crumble; a peace and joy that is surely supernatural, and always welcomed.

Hope keeps you going. It energizes you to have even more hope. How about a dream? Do you have a dream, or did you? Maybe it was crushed because of this injury. Maybe you just cannot do the things you used to. Maybe your energy level has plummeted and all you can do is think about "doing", then it's already a "done deal" because you're suddenly exhausted just thinking about it. What I do when that happens is ask God to give me strength to do what I need to do; to give me the energy and the wisdom to endure and to keep going. You can do that too if you like. He's always there, waiting for you to just ask. You can still dream your dream and plan for it coming to fruition. Make plans for your future and have hope, believing they will come true.

When we have a dream, we find ourselves with sudden energy just thinking about it. It lightens our mood and brightens our day. Just because we experience an injury and then have long-term effects of the aftermath, does not mean that life has stopped for us. It was just altered a bit. We need to have a new mindset, one that brings positivity, not negativity. We may just have to think outside the box in our circumstance and do what we can do, within the field of our dream. It may be a little different then we had originally imagined but it can still be fulfilling just the same.

When we have something placed within our hearts, something to do, someone to be, it excites us because it is a gift. We shouldn't brush it off as childish but rather embrace it because we're never too old to try. When we were formed in our mother's bellies, we were all, each and every one of us, being made special with unique gifts and talents all our own. Sure, we may have similarities to other people, with certain traits and temperaments, behaviors, as well as weaknesses but we are all fearfully and most wonderfully made "special". There is only one you! Be the best "you", you can be.

Let's think of our long-lost dreams again and awaken the zeal inside of us to find a way to somehow pursue them. Again, we can ask God's help in this. He knows how because He put those dreams inside our hearts in the first place. Surely, He can lead us to fulfilling them and in turn, fulfilling us. What hope and excitement for our future awaits us. When we think on these things, the pains and disappointments in life lose their power over us.

Everyone goes through something and grass is not always greener on the other side. It is all how we perceive things. When someone has hope they are able to smile in their trials. They are not as easily moved when things go wrong, and they will, because they are grounded in a Higher power that can bring good out of a bad.

If God can comfort, provide, protect, heal, defend, deliver, redeem and save us, surely, He can help us through this and any other difficult time in our lives. He is Lord Almighty and nothing, no not anything. is too hard for Him. Maybe we can't but God can. He has not brought you this far in life just to leave you hangin' at the face of your giant. You can overcome and conquer this through His love and strength that is made perfect through your trials of weakness. We all have these trials and we can all overcome and conquer them with His help. He is right there holding us up, even when we only think we are all alone. You need not be in despair through the turmoil of a brain injury, or any other life-changing event. You can experience hope and even find joy in your circumstance. So please, have hope and persevere through this. It will make a warrior out of you! I promise!

And we know that all things work together for good to them that love God, to them who are the called according to *his* purpose.
Romans 8:28 KJV

Finally, brothers and sisters, whatever is true, whatever is noble, whatever is right, whatever is pure, whatever is lovely, whatever is admirable—if anything is excellent or praiseworthy—think about such things.
Philippians 4:8 NIV

And he said unto me, My grace is sufficient for thee: for my strength is made perfect in weakness. Most gladly therefore will I rather glory in my infirmities, that the power of Christ may rest upon me.
2 Corinthians 12:9 KJV

A cheerful heart is good medicine, but a
crushed spirit dries up the bones.
Proverbs 17:22 NIV

Diet Does Matter

Life is busy and many of us are broke, or at least, broke minded. We are stressed and under even more stress, just thinking about what's for dinner, what's for lunch and what are we going to eat tomorrow. Some of us may take the "easy way" out, as we drive by, (or whoever is driving for that matter as some of us can't even drive yet from the brain injury fall-out) past a fast-food restaurant. We think, "dollar menu" as a choice for us and our family, only to find that over time, that "dollar menu" or "value meal" is really of no value at all in the long run, but just the opposite as the effects are felt in our health. What is the true value of a value meal? Think about it. If something costs only about a buck for a meat-like substance, and they still have to pay their employees, business expenses, and for the product in the first place, what is left? Is there any real nutritious food in it?

What is left is cheap disease-causing food as it is inflammatory causing to the core. Inflammation causes disease as it causes our bodies to go haywire. Every time you eat a buck's worth of inflammation, you are not saving anything as it is of no real value except satisfying an instant hunger craving. That so-called "value" will turn into a huge expense, at your expense.

I can't stress it enough about the importance of anti-inflammatories through natural means. Through our diet intake each day, we either contribute to inflammation and pain, or we treat it and reduce it, through what we eat and drink. So many of the foods today are a negative culprit in exasperating systems associated with inflammation. That being said, having a brain injury and dealing with the onslaught of symptoms, along with the challenging effects of learning to live with Post-Concussion Syndrome, our brains and therefore our bodies are already taxed with an inflammatory process going on. When we add to that, foods in our diet that cause additional inflammation, we have an overload of symptomatic problems developing throughout our bodily systems.

No wonder many of our uncomfortable complaints are pain, as in both headaches and also joint pain due to the adrenal glands being over taxed and completely exhausted, causing adrenal fatigue with a host of health issues and disease processes underway. Foods like white pastas, white rice, white flour, refined sugars, processed foods, and especially high-fructose corn syrup all cause inflammation in the body, setting the stage for disease. Stay away from them as much as possible.

High-fructose corn syrup is a cheap alternative sweetener, sometimes hidden with a name of "fructose-glucose syrup", that is added to so many food items including cereals, many breads, sodas, some yogurts and ice cream brands, snacks, syrups and sauces, even some canned goods, to give them that special sweetness. It is not only inflammation causing but also cancer causing, obesity, diabetes, and heart disease causing because it drives inflammation through the roof, which also sets you up for and makes worse auto-immune diseases.

Resveratrol, found in red wine is very beneficial for the body, especially when suffering from chronic pain and inflammation; although alcohol, if consumed, should only be drank in moderation, if at all depending upon your own personal health and beliefs. Liquor and spirits especially can place a burden on the liver as excess alcohol weakens liver function as well as disrupts the interaction between organs, causing inflammation. However, with that being said, if you are a casual drinker or say a consumer of wine with a meal, it is far better to drink a homemade wine as there will be less preservatives, if any at all. Red wine is best because it contains Resveratrol and Quercetin which have anti-oxidant and anti-inflammatory properties. Just think, learning to make home-made wine can turn into a new hobby for you, with the joys of "do it yourself" wine making. You will engage both your brain and your palate.

Some say, I myself included, that homemade wine helps with joint pain and overall stiffness. It's got to be the antioxidants and anti-inflammatories found naturally in the grapes. We can become connoisseurs of a delectable and delightful array of choices from the vast variety of red grape wines. We may find a liking to, or fancy a Merlot or perhaps a Malbec, or even a Cabernet Sauvignon. This could be a good thing! We could tell our friends it's research for our auto-immune disorder. Just don't go overboard.

Inflammation is very destructive to the human body, which has been given to you to take care of by giving it the best nutrition as possible, so it may run efficiently and heal appropriately.

Question: If you had an amazing sports car like say a Ferrari, a Lamborghini, Porsche, Jaguar, Corvette or a Camaro, or any other particular car you fancy, would you give it the cheapest watered-down gasoline or fuel? Heck no! So, why would you feed yourself cheap alternatives rather than real food? Is it okay for your body to breakdown—but not your dream car? You are precision made! Why intentionally then would you "break" yourself down?

Inflammation comes in all types, from many sources: injury, environment, chemicals, insecticides (neuro toxins), parasites, infections, mold, fungus and "food" sources.

It is absolutely paramount to read all food labels for a list of ingredients; the less in any product, the better. If you purchase a product that has a long list of ingredients that you can't even recognize the names of or what they stand for, along with a lengthy shelf-life date, then you are buying a chemical concoction for means of ingestion to satisfy hunger, of "supposed nutrition" in the name of "food", but without any real nutritional value, leaving your body starving still for nutrition. With items that mention "food-like" or "cheese-like" you are buying plastics to ingest. When buying juice cocktail, juice beverage, etc., you are really buying a disease process in a can or bottle. These are either made of plastics and/or sugar (high-fructose corn syrup); both of which are not meant for human consumption as they alter the cells within your body causing inflammation and diseases, such as diabetes and cancer.

Now when someone has a brain injury, they need real nutrition, food with a nutritional value to help the body maintain homeostasis (proper functioning and repair), as there is a big healing process going on and also great inflammation already started due to the injury. We must not add to the inflammation by a poor diet and inadvertently cause more damage to the body coupled with an impaired healing process. The human body can only take so much to what is thrown at it. That being said, the human body is also quite capable of great healing and repair, as well as growth, through proper diet. It is all in the food and what we call nutrition. You know that old saying, "You are what you eat"? Well it is true. You are. If you eat garbage, then garbage will result through disease, poor healing and poor recovery.

Your brain has much on its plate with caring for and orchestrating all your bodily functions and systems, enabling them to run properly. When it is damaged, as well as when it is not, feed it with excellence. Feed your body the brain food it needs. You would not feed a human being dog or cat food. Although we can all feed a healthier diet to our beloved pets through "real" people foods (meats and certain veggies, some fruits—not junk), but that is a topic for another discussion so please do your research. The point is, why not feed our brain, an injured brain, brain food!

We have all most likely heard by now how bad sugar is for you. You have probably heard that too much can cause diabetes but still you may not be concerned. You may have heard that sugar feeds cancer cells and causes them to proliferate, to multiply rapidly. But have you heard, other than reading it above, that sugar also adds to inflammation? Eating added sugar to your diet, (including soda or pop), refined carbohydrates (white flours, pasta, white rice, white potatoes, crackers, etc.) and gluten will increase your inflammatory markers as they are proinflammatory; promotes inflammation.

Ever notice after eating a high carb meal, sugar and gluten filled, that you are about to completely crash? I mean you could suddenly wonder if you now have narcolepsy (a sleep disorder) because you are having trouble keeping your eyes open, even if it is not anywhere near your bedtime, and your about to fall asleep standing up. Your body is reacting and can't keep up with the overload—so it's shutting you down in order to do its job of keeping your heart beating, your respiration going, and all the intricate things it does as it is attempting to pump out the correct amounts of hormones and enzymes to handle such an onslaught. Phew, that is tiresome work! No wonder you are suddenly fatigued to the max, exhausted and have to sleep, NOW!

When it comes to hunger, sugar cravings, and gluten intolerance, there in addition can be, especially due to a brain injury which could lead to damage to the hypothalamus, a "leptin" imbalance (hormones that regulate energy, balanced by inhibiting hunger) within the body, causing further sugar cravings and also a "ghrelin" imbalance (the hunger hormone), because they both act on receptors within the hypothalamus. Evidence may be being overweight and still have food cravings, especially sugar type foods. This then leads to "lectins" (sugar binding proteins) binding carbohydrates and attaching to cells, further promoting inflammation as they are proinflammatory, presenting with immunotoxicity (causing adverse effects in the immune system), are neurotoxic (adversely effects the peripheral nervous system) and cytotoxic (toxic to living cells); plus, can also further disrupt endocrine function which is not good for an already compromised endocrine system and now negatively engages the immune system. Here we have three major systems within the body negatively affected by lectins: the endocrine system, immune system and the nervous system.

Let's not even get started on "GMO's" and the damaging effects to the human body caused by the toxicity and highly durable lectins from an "enhanced" and "tampered" food source. You are playing a game of Russian Roulette if you consume GMO's because the trigger with the disease filled bullet will go off, right into your cells. Now, that enormously big, perfectly looking ripe piece of fruit no longer has the appeal of being healthy, does it! Monsanto (an agricultural company bought by Bayer) is right up there with Big Pharma, testing their poisons on an ant farm, us humans, but on a scale that consists of the entire planet we live and breathe on, called earth!

Balance is everything. When there is, for instance, an imbalance of Omega-6 fatty acids to Omega-3's, there is an increase in leptin (leptin resistance) and also insulin resistance, affecting your food intake, metabolism and blood sugar levels increasing the risk for obesity and Diabetes. Some foods that can decrease leptin resistance and lower insulin levels are unprocessed oatmeal, grapefruit, lean proteins (grass-fed is best), green tea, fish, eggs, broccoli (rich in Vit. C), almonds, fruits and vegetables, beans, olive oil, Turmeric, sesame seeds, and Spirulina. They will help lower the levels while increasing your metabolism.

Now since lectins are abundant in certain food sources such as gluten containing foods and grain such as wheat, (which includes oils made with grain—corn oil, condiments and dressings), raw legumes, dairy (if animal was fed grain rather than grass as a diet) and some vegetables known as "nightshades": tomatoes, eggplant, peppers and potatoes, they are however, not digestible. Because we cannot digest lectins, our bodies instead produce antibodies to them, which in turn can make these certain foods intolerable to us and our gut, especially if we have had a change within our immune system, as in an injury causing inflammation and also the onset on an autoimmune disease, especially inflammatory bowel disease and Crohn's disease, because of the extremely sensitive atmosphere of the bowel.

Now even if you do not suffer from any type of bowel disease, the bowel can and most likely is affected by any other type of auto-immune disease or disorder that you are dealing with, and you may already be noticing some differences in your bowel habits as far as frequency and consistency. All these changes should be brought to the attention of who is treating you, preferably a naturopath or a practitioner that specializes in a holistic approach to medicine and healing. We want to feel better. Heck, we want to get better, not worse. Am I right?

With the right diet, by cleaning up the diet and the utilizing natural treatments as well as living in a clean environment, as there are many toxins in our environment, we may be able to introduce some foods back into our diets slowly, depending on what typically bothers us and our immune system, with regard to our overall health. We need to make sure our bodies are getting enough real nutrition with enough vitamins and minerals to thrive, such vitamins B-12, C and D, also zinc and magnesium. So, don't freak out if your healthcare provider suggests that you stop eating peppers or tomatoes, at least temporarily as the gut lining may very well be sensitive to these, if they think it could be causing your painful symptoms, because their advice is meant to help you feel better. Right there can be cause for a "freak out" for me because I just love them, especially jalapenos! I personally, can eat them at almost every meal. They are a staple in my little world. Sometimes though, for our health, we may need to change things up a little bit, at least for a short while if need be.

So, if we suffer from or have recently been diagnosed with an auto-immune disease or disorder, when these "lectins" enter our bodies, they will stimulate an immune response, usually causing stiffness, swelling and pain as well as disturbance in our gut, causing a leaky gut (bloating, gas, cramps), leading to intestinal permeability, where nutrients aren't absorbed properly and substances leak into the bloodstream. This is a huge problem because the gut is our biggest immune system organ. When lectins affect the wall of the gut, the intestines, there is a huge inflammatory response as the body moves into defense mode to attack the invaders. Enter, unrefined coconut oil to help your gut repair and heal as well as fermented foods to add in good bacteria that is so beneficial to your gut.

Now, not all lectin responses in the body are bad, as there are beneficial and health promoting lectins that are important to achieve basic functions within the body, but there needs to be balance, not imbalance. Additionally, the negative effects can be greatly reduced and quite possibly be reversed with a change in diet by adding a number of fruits and vegetables along with coconut oil (unrefined) and fermented foods. We are talking about a variety here.

What Helps Both Brain & Body

Bloodwork is essential not only for brain injured individuals to check for fluctuations and imbalances in hormones, vitamins and minerals, enzymes, blood cell counts, inflammatory makers, thyroid function, endocrine function, et cetera but is also important for those suffering from inflammation. Inflammation can have an effect on vitamin D levels, causing deficiency, in that it is a consequence of chronic inflammation as well as a contributing cause. Though Vit. D can be absorbed through the skin under sunlight, it is not enough when it comes to inflammation. Supplementation must be added in addition to a clean healthy diet especially if you're are fighting an auto-immune response—disease or disorder.

If you are Vit. D deficient and have a leaky gut in response to gluten, your ability to even absorb the fat soluble Vit. D in greatly diminished, which just brings you around in an endless loop of inflammation. In this case, we must get the bloodwork, stop eating gluten containing foods and up our Vit. D intake to help battle this huge inflammatory process going on. Vit. D will strengthen our immune system and help it to not attack our own bodies. In order to best regulate how much Vit. D you should be taking, first have your levels checked and depending on deficiency amounts, your care provider can best offer you the correct dosage needed, which may range from 2000 units, up to and between 5000-8000 units. The range is big, therefore, check first and have follow-up bloodwork taken to check results along with monitoring your inflammatory symptoms.

When it comes to food and the diet of every individual, especially when healing from an injury such as a brain injury, nutrition is of tremendous importance to help the body and brain heal. Certain foods are packed with nutrient dense nutrition; amino acids, anti-oxidants, anti-inflammatories, omegas, probiotics, et cetera and they are a powerhouse of not only fuel for your body, but all the extras your body and brain need to facilitate the healing process of tissue and nerve repair.

Probiotics, easily found in fermented foods such as sauerkraut, yogurts in varying degrees, kefir and my personal favorite Kombucha, are not just for a healthy gut, no they also indirectly enhance brain function as well as immune function. Kombucha, which also has enzymes beneficial for arthritic pain as they are anti-inflammatory in nature, comes in many flavors so if you are suffering from an autoimmune disorder, guess what, it comes in tart cherry which helps with pain relief as well. Yeah, double whammy! I just love it!

There is a biochemical signaling between the nervous system within the digestive tract known as the enteric nervous system, and the central nervous system which includes the brain that connects the gut and the brain together, called the gut/brain axis with the primary connection between the two by the vagus nerve; the tenth cranial nerve being the longest nerve within the autonomic nervous system. Besides the vagus nerve having many functions including motor and sensory, it also interacts with parasympathetic control of the lungs, heart and the digestive tract, supplying innervation, distribution of nerves, to the gastro-intestinal tract—the gut. The gut is sometimes referred to as the second brain. Like the saying goes, "You are what you eat." Not only can we tell physically if we eat the wrong things, for instance noticing oncoming headaches, body aches, bloating, sluggishness, even extreme fatigue if gluten is a problem for someone, but also the "feel good" foods like chocolate that increase levels of serotonin and stimulates the release of dopamine. Yum! No wonder I feel so good after eating chocolate; so, bring on the chocolate!

The gut also produces many neurotransmitters, much as the brain does, that affect our mood like serotonin, gamma-aminobutyric acid (GABA-relieves anxiety) and yes, dopamine. I don't know about you but I'm thinking chocolate again; okay maybe the dark chocolate because it contains less sugar and is better for you with these amazing benefits.

Serotonin is that "happy" neurotransmitter that has the opposite effect when levels are low. In fact, low levels of serotonin are linked to depression and memory problems. We don't want that. We already have enough on our plate with all that's happening since the injury. Right? Besides the obvious of being a happy and well-being neurotransmitter, serotonin also is an important neurotransmitter, transmitting messages between nerve cells, active in constricting smooth muscles and also is a precursor for melatonin; helping the body regulate sleep and wake cycles—regulating the internal clock.

Serotonin impacts the nervous system, which then plays a role in emotions, motor and cognitive function, appetite and also autonomic functions (heart and respiratory rates, digestion, pupillary response, urination and yes, even sexual responses and arousal). All this is controlled by the autonomic nervous system and is regulated, now get this—by the hypothalamus. There it is, part of that connection. So, if there is damage, there is a disconnect. However, with that being said, the serotonin that is used in the brain, must be produced in the brain, because it does not cross the blood brain barrier. Because serotonin relays signals between the nerve cells, it plays a very important key role within the central nervous system and overall functioning of the body, especially the gut; the gastrointestinal tract. There are crucial links between serotonin and liver regeneration, breast milk production, bone metabolism (ossification-new bone formation) and cell division. Serotonin has such an impact, it both directly and indirectly influences brain cells and bodily function.

One thing to note that is also controlled autonomically is the "fight-or-flight" response that so many of us brain injured individuals deal with, sometimes on a daily basis. Sometimes it just lingers for years, past the acute phase of being diagnosed with a TBI (Traumatic Brain Injury) and even way through some extended period of time living with PCS (Post-

Concussion Syndrome). That disconnect from damage in the brain, in the hypothalamus, directly affects the link the brain shares with the gut as serotonin is also produced there. But, is the body responding accordingly to the correct levels it needs to function properly and virtually symptom free?

- Something to note, just because you may have lower levels of serotonin, taking 5-HTP, a by-product of L-tryptophan (amino acid used in synthesis of proteins), increases the production of serotonin which may be beneficial in most cases—except, if you are taking anti-depressants! *** If you have been diagnosed with depression and are already taking anti-depressant medication, do Not take 5-HTP because some drugs also raise serotonin levels, causing very serious side-effects including shivering, anxiety and also heart problems. Also make sure to check for any drug interaction!

If you are not on any anti-depressant medication, serotonin may be of help to you in the form of 5-HTP. Check with your physician first. 5-HTP is helpful for insomnia and sleep disorders, anxiety, migraines, headaches, Fibromyalgia, and is used in people suffering from seizures, Parkinson's as well as ADHD (Attention Deficit Hyperactivity Disorder—many times diet also helps). 5-HTP is also used for and is helpful in minor depression and feelings of melancholy, just not if already taking an anti-depressant!

The human body is absolutely amazing in what it can do, not only physically on the outside to which we can all perceive, but also internally within each body system, and also emotionally as foods can also play a role in one's emotional state of being by having an effect on dopamine and serotonin levels in the brain. The human body is capable of restoring homeostasis; that is to say, a healthy state of being.

Okay, back to chocolate, I mean, dopamine. Since dopamine also boosts levels of serotonin, as does chocolate in itself, it is thought to relieve stress. So, that is why people love chocolate so much; people are stressed. With the plight of dealing with additional stressors of PCS symptoms and now auto-immune disorders, we have become not only stressed and more stressed but also inflamed with a ton of inflammation going on, that only seems to cause, you guessed it, more stress. So, bring out the chocolate. You can say, "Honey, can you go to the store and get me some chocolate? I have to eat it because it is good and good for me." They may respond, "Yeah right!" Seriously, just don't eat too much. You don't want to need to be concerned about your glucose levels next.

Besides the compound phenylethylamine found in chocolate that is responsible for stimulating the brain to release dopamine, there is also present tyramine, derived from the amino acid tyrosine which also has similar dopamine producing effects. Ironically or should I say oddly enough, there are more concentrations present in white chocolate rather than in the presumed dark, though dark chocolate contains antioxidants which can help reduce inflammation and lower blood pressure, not found in white or milk chocolate. Now get this, according to Georgia Health Sciences University, the brain will produce dopamine even if you are only "thinking" about chocolate. Now, that is guilt free!

See how powerful our brains are. We all should be careful what we think as thoughts can play a role in our moods and therefore health. So, whenever a bad or negative thought comes to mind, you can kick it out along with the downcast feelings associated with it and think about chocolate instead. It is the limbic system in full response acting as a mild anti-depressant gearing up a feel-good emotional response. Although some may argue that the mood-altering substances found in chocolate are too low if consumed in normal amounts and that it is actually the fats and carbohydrates in the form of sugar that lead to a "comfort food" craving, there usually still is a boost in mood, if only temporary. So, perhaps thinking about it will be enough, or not; okay maybe just a bite. Personally, I like mine melted with fruit such as strawberries and pineapple dipped in. Can I get a "Yum"?

Now, besides dark chocolate having the benefits of antioxidants to help reduce inflammation, it also helps increase arterial blood flow reducing blood clot formation as our moods are overall, even if only temporarily, boosted along with brain chemicals. This antioxidant benefit is due to the flavonoid compounds that are found not only in dark chocolate but also in natural cocoa that is not treated with alkali through Dutch processing, (code name-Dutch cocoa). Once cocoa is treated with alkali, most of the beneficial flavonoid compounds are removed.

Again, if you do choose to partake in eating chocolate, don't over indulge too much because an excess of it will lead to too much dopamine in the limbic system causing negative responses including paranoia. Just think, "Paranoid from too much chocolate"? As for Me? Never! But, moderation is definitely the key, as with anything. Too much of a good thing can backfire and turn bad. Even chocolate. Hmmmm....Now, that is something to ponder on.

One thing is for certain, you can never have too much hope, or faith in a higher power to help you get through this or anything else life deals to you. Then, you will be better equipped to help others going through the same or similar circumstances. I surely say this from experience. As much as I love, love, love chocolate, it does not satisfy life quite like the sweet aroma of a joy filled life, trusting in my Savior.

So, what about if you do not like chocolate? Yes, these people do exist, my older daughter being one of them. Crazy huh? I can't even imagine a world without chocolate. Maybe I like it a little too much. Perhaps my extra portion of liking chocolate didn't get passed down to her—poor girl. Am I a bad parent for not passing down the love of chocolate? Lord knows I tried. I would continually buy her chocolate at different times during the years, but she really never enjoyed my gift to her. She truly does not even realize what she is missing. Now, if it was steak, we would have a winner for her. Me on the other hand, if I miss just a week without chocolate, I would probably go crazy. I may even have a "freak out" session in my own head, to everyone's amazement of what all the "hubba" was about. It's about chocolate, man! Can't anyone understand the passion? I honestly am so thankful every time I eat it. I can't believe that something so good is going into my mouth. I have my moment of tranquility with each bite. With that, as I'm sure I'm making some pretty amusing facial expressions, people probably already think I'm crazy. Uh, no—just enjoying my chocolate! If you're with me, maybe I'll share. I mean, I don't want to be selfish now.

Other food ideas for dopamine filled bliss are Omega-3 rich fish such as salmon, eggs, fruits & vegetables—for instance bananas, almonds, walnuts and other nuts & seeds--unprocessed and non-GMO, grass-fed with no antibiotics, hormones or drugs-- chicken, turkey & beef (expensive I know but worth your health), because "non"-grass-fed beef is inflammatory, as is non-grass-fed animal sources for yogurts & cheese; regular dairy is inflammatory. When purchasing yogurt, look at the label for sugar content as well as protein, we want less sugar and more protein along with the choice of more probiotics. Don't forget to eat at regular mealtimes to avoid a crash and mood swings. Additionally, add some physical activity and exercise to your daily routine.

There are many foods to avoid and even remove from your diet if you are suffering from an auto-immune disorder, even if it is brought about from an initial brain injury. Think of it this way, the damage is done, and the inflammation has already wreaked havoc on your body. So now, your diet along with your environment comes into play as it will affect your health further. You will notice more and more stiffness, swelling, aches and pains in the joints as well as possibly the muscles and bones. Because there was such an inflammatory process going on with the initial blow, your diet, what you eat each and every diet will have an impact further on your well-being.

Not only is it crucial to remove completely high fructose corn syrup from your diet, but also refined flour, refined grain products and refined sugar, which are all highly processed and chemically produced. Keeping these in your diet will no doubt have a very negative effect on your body, your inflammation, your healing and also your overall health; you need your health in order to be free from disease. Now keep in mind that we all need to start a habit of reading food labels and don't think for a second that "low fat" will help you in any way because guess what, more sugar is added to the products to help with the taste.

Ever wonder what makes foods last so long, and be so soft, such as in breads and some baked goods, and also make them taste so good and even addicting? It is the unnatural chemical processes and concoctions of additives used. This is killing your immune system! Next question. Ever wonder why so many people are exhibiting symptoms of an auto-immune disorder or disease these days? I mean it is everywhere you go. You hear it all the time. It is due to our foods, heavily, as they are a companion source of disease. I say companion source because if we just clean up our diets, we will not only feel so much better, we will also exhibit less and less inflammatory symptoms.

When we come down with an auto-immune disease, there is a ton of inflammation going on in the body and the body therefore cannot do its job correctly or efficiently to keep us healthy. It starts to talk to us through some form of stiffness and discomfort; but do we listen? Our body then starts to scream at us with heavy fatigue as it attempts to have us rest so it can try to heal, but because of the disconnects and chaos inside, it attacks us instead, thinking our good guy cells are the enemy. Swelling of joints start, more stiffness, locking fingers and toes, then pain, pain and more pain. Redness can appear at different points on our bodies, including our face which everybody sees, depending on which of the many auto-immune diseases start.

Somehow, we are caught off-guard, oblivious that our own diets can be the culprit to our down turn in our health. We may be still caught up with the many symptoms of our Traumatic Brain Injury and the debilitating effects of Post-Concussion Syndrome to pay attention. So now, when this new "player" joins the game in our life, we're like, "What-what?" "Auto-immune?"

Maybe we thought it was just hereditary. Maybe we still think it's just hereditary as we keep eating inflammatory foods that our family always made and ate, though making it worse and worse. Then we go for bloodwork and receive the shock of our lives. There it is, in black and white. Yet, we may still think, "How can this be?" We may think our diets don't seem bad. But diet, along with any other culprit of inflammation, is continually causing and maintaining an inflammatory process; keeping us inflamed.

Oh, What to Do, What to Do

It can be overwhelming, boy don't I know, when it comes to eating and eating healthy; especially with getting everybody on the same page as you are. First of all, you had a brain injury and are already overwhelmed; thank you very much! Now, we have to add food into the mix; and meal planning? Say it isn't so! Let me share something with you. Food, stresses me out! I mean, I can eat it if it suddenly appears in front of me. I'm actually quite delighted whenever that happens, which is not too often.

But to have myself in charge of the "meal thing", that's another story. The funny thing is, is that it never used to be that way. In fact, I used to like, bordering on love, to cook. I would even have holiday dinners at my house and relished the fact of large groups of people, I call family, attending. But now, oh no! Not any more. If I knew twenty or thirty some odd people were about to come over for dinner, even if I had plenty of time in advance to plan it, I would just freak out. I get overwhelmed just thinking about it now. Maybe I should think of chocolate instead—yay dopamine! So now, all my extra plates used for those dinners sit in my hutch and wait for me to occasionally grab one and eat off of it. I'm sure if they had feelings, all the other plates in there would be jealous.

As for recipes? I need to have very short ones that I can look at several times during preparation of a meal. If it has too many ingredients, well, it's too long for me. I can even open the refrigerator door in search of an idea and feel panic. That is when I remind myself to just breathe. Breathe in four deep breaths and then exhale out four. Four to five works, but you get the picture.

I call to mind a Scripture verse from the book of Exodus in the Bible, verse 33:14, that helps immensely; "My presence shall go with you and I will give you rest." That way I remember, I am not alone in my struggle, wherever I'm at and whatever I'm doing, even if it is only over meal preparation. It helps me to know that God is in control and He is bigger than my problems and struggles in life that can so easily overwhelm me. He is Sovereign over all things and has it all, including me and including you. I also remind myself that "No weapon formed against me shall prosper"—Isaiah 54:17, including any stress or anxiety-filled moments, or my pain, disorder, illness, or injury! God is surely bigger!

I need to just rest in Him, stay focused on Him and not look at my problems or difficulties; because when we start to look down and see all our problems and worries, we begin to sink. We feel the sinking in our gut. But, if we can stay focused on the Lord, trusting that He has this, we will find that we can keep going in a forward flow and all will be fine. What I end up finding is a peace in my heart that quiets my anxious soul, and you will too. This is a peace that surpasses all understanding, in all things, even when it comes to food and meal preparation.

Brain/Body Foods & Herbs

That Fight Inflammation

• **W**alnuts, **A**lmonds & **P**ecans—are all high in unsaturated fats to help reduce inflammation and lubricate the joints, keeping them moving smoothly. Nuts, though they are of the nightshade family and can bother some people with a lectin sensitivity, are high in fiber, vitamins, minerals, protein and phytosterols—capable of lowering LDL, "bad", cholesterol by 14%. They are also a great source of Omega-3 fatty acids which is perfect to decrease the C-Reactive protein. Walnuts are said to inhibit the production of neurotransmitters that are responsible for increased pain and inflammation.

• **O**mega-**3** Fatty Acid rich foods are very beneficial in inflammatory diseases, heart diseases and auto-immune diseases. The

Omega-3's are ALA (Alpha-linolenic Acid)—plant based found in green leafy vegetables, chia seeds, walnuts and flaxseeds, EPA (Eicosapentaenoic Acid)—found in oily fish, krill oil and algae oil, and DHA (Docosahexaenoic Acid) also found in oily fish, krill and algae oils.

Omega-3's are essential fatty acids that your body does not make, but that you must consume through your diet. It is recommended by the American Heart Association to consume 2 or more, 3.5 ounce servings of fish per week. If you suffer from heart disease, anxiety, depression or cancer, higher amounts of consumptions are recommended.

It is possible to be Omega-3 deficient if suffering from fatigue, memory problems, poor circulation, dry skin, heart problems, mood swings and even depression. But it can be difficult to consume that much fish each week, so supplementation is another route to go to receive Omega-3's into your body.

Adding Omega-3's to your diet either through food or supplementation will help with reducing inflammation, fight auto-immune diseases, improve your heart health, lower your cancer risk, improve your sleep quality, improve your mood and mental state by reducing anxiety and depression while stabilizing behaviors, support healthy bones and joints by enhancing the effect of vitamin D, aid in skin and eye support, slow aging, fight menstrual pain and is neuroprotective in fighting against cognitive decline.

Since Omega-3's are so good at reducing inflammation, and since a brain injury causes great inflammation in the brain, (that affects the entire body with miscommunication, mixed and missed signals, potentially causing more inflammation), by adding them into an anti-inflammatory diet they will help with the effects of inflammation and reduce it. It is absolutely paramount to make sure you are getting enough Omega-3's in your diet.

Additionally, Omega-3's are helpful not only in managing an auto-immune disorder, they are also linked to a decreased risk of an auto-immune disorder and improvement in overall symptoms. There is a protective effect that goes on when consuming Omega-3's, especially within the first year of life, which is super important for babies. If you have not added it to you diet yet, don't wait. There is no better time than the present especially if you have suffered from a concussion or traumatic brain injury.

• **Hemp Seeds & Hempseed Oil**— Hemp seeds are high in protein, supplying amino acids needed for your growth, health and repair/maintenance within the body. The protein from hemp contains all 20 amino acids including the 9 essential that is needed for homeostasis with 65% of the protein being made up of the globulin protein Edestin, which aids in digestion and is the backbone of cell's DNA— making DNA repair possible. When DNA is damaged whether through radiation, toxins, injury or disease, including many discussed within this book, Edestin protein found in hemp seeds is a major factor in DNA repair as cells will use this protein to correct the damage. In addition, Edestin also produces antibodies vital to maintaining a healthy immune system. Aren't our bodies amazing in what it can do with the right nutrition?

Hempseed oil has been known as "Nature's most perfectly balanced oil" due to the balanced ratio of Omegas in relation to essential fatty acids and is recommended for long-term healthy nutrition with its rich supply of antioxidants, vitamins and minerals. Hempseed oil is best used as a flavor enhancer to food recipes before serving and not during the cooking process as it will break down to trans-fat when heated; so, don't cook with it but enjoy it added to favorite recipes. Once opened it is best stored in the refrigerator.

Hemp seeds are very easy to add to your diet as they can be eaten in a variety of ways from a spoonful, to nice additions to yogurts and smoothies. They are also wonderful topped on a salad or sprinkled on a number of foods; even dopamine rich chocolate. Now we're talkin'.

• **C**hlorella— Both Chlorella and its close relative Spirulina are excellent choices in helping your body rid itself of the heavy metal toxicity that accompanies the "American diet" as well as environment hazards we are so often exposed to. It works much like Moringa in the sense that they are a nutritious detox, that rids the body of toxins through elimination via your bowel, so it's best to start off slowly. Accumulation of these toxins cause detrimental health issues, relating to auto-immune disorders and also making them worse. Detoxing the body is one of the best things you can do—then replace with wholefood and healing nutrition.

Chlorella is a natural supplement that boosts your energy levels while it also supports fat loss. It is considered a superfood with phytonutrients, beta-carotene, amino acids, B-complex vitamins, magnesium, potassium, biotin, iron, zinc, protein, and more. It supports hormonal function, cardiovascular health, lowers blood pressure and cholesterol. Chlorella is ranked one of the top 10 nutrient dense foods, even more than spinach, broccoli, kale or other greens per gram.

Chlorella is so important in detoxifying the body of heavy metals, even ones you may not think of such as from vaccines, mercury tooth fillings, radiation, even chemotherapy, that it can also be used as a proactive approach and in turn support your immune system making it healthier as it helps natural killer cell activities.

- **Reishi Mushroom (Ganoderma)**— Known as the "king" of herbs has so many beneficial and healing properties because it actually oxygenates your cells and makes the body more alkaline and resistant to disease processes. We most likely have all heard by now that disease grows in an acidic environment. Ganoderma, the other name for Reishi mushroom, counteracts that and brings the body back to a healthy state.

Ganoderma is a true superfood that not only fights cancer, improves liver detoxification, but also boosts immunity by balancing the immune system as it is an immune system modulator. When the immune system is sluggish, it boosts it. If the immune system is overactive, as in the case of auto-immune disorders, Ganoderma slows it down and brings it back into balance to do its job of protecting the body, not fighting it or harming it. The Reishi mushroom (Ganoderma) has medicinal properties and healing capabilities which are highly anti-inflammatory in nature and is also linked to longevity, mental clarity along with improved immune function.

Ganoderma helps us to handle the negative effects of stress such as fatigue, hormonal imbalances, damaged blood vessels and the resulting increased inflammation through its antioxidant abilities, allowing the body to strengthen its defenses against inflammation, cancer, heart disease, infections, digestive problems, viruses, sleep disorders, skin disorders, anxiety and depression as well as auto-immune diseases, allergies and more.

How is this possible? Because Ganoderma (Reishi mushroom) works as an immune adaptogen. It works to restore the body back to homeostasis, back to health. It acts as a normalizer, regulating cellular functions and bodily systems, including endocrine, immune, digestive, cardiovascular and the central nervous system. Ganoderma is also said to have the ability to stimulate brain neurons. Yeah! Just what we need after a brain injury. So, bring it! Now, doesn't that sound like the king of herbs to do all that? It sure does! With its ability to reduce inflammation, aches, stiffness, pain, infections, digestive issues, and allergies all the while improving energy and mental clarity as well as increasing mood, it is a "must have" in the kitchen for the many suffering from auto-immune disorders.

You can add Reishi mushroom (Ganoderma) to your diet through tincture, extract, powder, tea and even coffee. Say what? Coffee you say? Yes, through a healthy blend of gourmet Arabic coffee beans with Ganoderma, the Reishi mushroom, in such a process as to supply the herbal health benefits, it is not only delicious, but smooth tasting as well. (There is a link in the back of this book on how to get yours...under "important links".) Ganoderma has 16 types of amino acids, 7 of which are essential and to think that we can combat the usual negative effects of regular coffee, which is acidic to the body, with healthy coffee which is alkaline, is absolutely amazing. It is a coffee lover's dream!

• **Chaga Mushroom Tea**—supports the immune system with immune system boosting ingredients and is also anti-oxidant in nature. Much like Ganoderma (Reishi mushroom), Chaga boosts the immune system when needed and slows it down when overactive as it is also adaptogenic; stabilizing and promoting homeostasis. Chaga also supports the blood vessels and helps with neuropathy and pain. Chaga additionally normalizes blood pressure and cholesterol levels, protects against DNA damage, supports gastrointestinal health and soothes ulcers. Chaga also has antiviral properties and fights against skin blemishes. It can be purchased already ground in bulk tea form. It is best to let Chaga steep for 30 minutes before drinking, for full extraction of the medicinal components. It's a great idea to cover your cup of tea while steeping to keep warm.

• **Unrefined Coconut Oil** (cold-pressed fresh coconut, to maintain the antioxidant and anti-inflammatory benefits)—Benefits include improved brain function, stimulation of metabolism, lowers risk for heart disease, has antibacterial, antifungal, antiviral and antimicrobial properties as well as boosts immune system with its anti-inflammatory properties. Adding coconut oil to your diet as well as skin care is one of the best things you can do. You can cook with it as it does not break down like other oils, nor does it interfere with thyroid function. In fact, it supports it.

Coconut oil is fantastic in coffee and a great way to get a spoonful into your diet. If you're not a fan of the coconut taste, refined (made from dried coconut, then steamed) coconut oil has a neutral taste without the coconut smell.

Coconut oil is one of the best alternative energy sources of fuel for your brain and malfunctioning brain cells as it supports brain function and health. Remember the brain gut connection discussed earlier? Coconut oil is perfect for your gut as it helps heal it, aids in digestion, helps shed excess body fat, and lowers the inflammation within your gut; which is beneficial for inflammatory bowel diseases such as Crohn's.

• **O**lives and **O**live **O**il—The polyphenols in olives have been shown to lower levels of the C-Reactive Protein, which is a marker for inflammation within the body.

• **G**oji **B**erries—are a high fiber, high antioxidant superfood with 20 different vitamins and minerals offering benefits ranging from weight management, better digestion, boost in energy levels and aids stamina, reduces fatigue, increases quality sleep, increases mental acuity and focus, reduces depression and anxiety, reduces blood glucose levels, regulates cholesterol levels, protects skin and eyes, lowers inflammation and more. Wow! They are power packed! Goji berries also contain protein ranging between 4 to 12 grams, which is perfect when we are trying to get that little extra protein in (you know what I mean if you have constant food struggles with kids—Phew!)

Goji berries can help boost your immune system function with its high levels of nutrients and antioxidants, which will ultimately help with inflammation and the corresponding stiffness, swelling and associated pain. However, they are considered to be of the nightshade family which can be proinflammatory for the gut and some auto-immune disorders as they do contain lectins despite their small size; monitor for any sensitivity to lectins if eating these. If you already have a leaky gut, heal your gut first. Goji berries even supply more beta-carotene than carrots and more iron than spinach—which will also help with an iron deficiency! Other benefits of goji berries are liver detoxification, stabilizing blood sugar levels, boosting moods while offering feelings of well-being, and also boosts fertility and libido. You probably want to go grab your mate and go get some, don't you? I'm talking about goji berries; what were you just thinking? Hey now, easy on those goji berries.

• **M**oringa **O**leifera— Moringa is a highly nutritious superfood with powerful anti-inflammatory, antioxidant and protective properties helpful in quality health. Moringa is nutrient packed with vitamins, minerals, amino acids, and omegas, supporting health while treating and often times preventing such diseases as diabetes, anemia, heart disease, liver disease, skin and digestive issues and also eases arthritic pain with its anti-inflammatory properties.

Moringa additionally supports brain health and cognitive function with its antioxidant and neuro enhancing activities and is also being used for Alzheimer's. Moringa's high content of vitamins C and E fight oxidation that leads to neuro degeneration while improving brain function. Moringa is actually able to normalize the neurotransmitters, serotonin, dopamine and noradrenaline in the brain, improving mood, memory, and mental health—making it beneficial for depression, organ function, and also plays a role in how we react to responses to various stimuli such as stress and pleasure.

Moringa additionally has antibacterial, antimicrobial and antifungal properties that have been effective in helping fight infections and strains of bacteria as well as beneficial in wound healing.

It comes in a powdered form that makes it easy to drink by adding it to water, smoothies or even drink as a tea. If you are not used to eating rich "greens" in your diet, start off slow with a ½ teaspoon to begin with as the highly beneficial, and nutrient dense "green food" can act much like chlorella at first giving a slight laxative effect in attempts of your body trying to clear itself of toxins and heavy metals from chemicals, pesticides, processed foods, and certain sea foods such as bottom feeders. You can increase the amount as your body gets accustomed to this dense superfood nutrition.

• **Tart Cherries or Tart Cherry Juice**—is known to reduce pain and inflammation, including soreness from exercises. Tart cherry juice can easily be added to smoothies and dried tart cherries can be added to yogurt or cereal; plus, it conveniently comes in some Kombuchas, or can be added to homemade ones.

• Grapes—are known to have anti-inflammatory properties and is also packed with anti-oxidants. Red grapes contain Resveratrol, a compound group of polyphenols that act as an anti-oxidant protecting the body against damage and lowers the risk of heart disease and cancer. This is what makes red wine so good for you, especially homemade. Grapes also help with Parkinson's disease, Alzheimer's and Raynaud's Syndrome (especially grapes seed extract to improve blood circulation), which is common in arthritis and Fibromyalgia. Grapes can even be frozen for a tasty treat anytime!

• Turmeric—Oh wonderful Turmeric! Turmeric is a compound of curry, with its active ingredient Curcumin and is widely known for its overall health benefits and anti-inflammatory properties as well as protective properties against cancer and tumor growth. It helps with pain and inflammation, reduces tumors, is an anti-oxidant and is also neuroprotective. It comes in root form but can also be purchased dried to easily add to foods and also comes in a tincture form for stronger potency, (You can even make your own tincture by shredding the root in a mason jar filled with an extraction medium such as vodka, letting it sit for approximately 4-6 weeks. A dropperful can be added to food or water.) ***Be sure to add fresh ground peppercorn for increased absorption by a whopping 2000%***

• **Q**uercetin rich foods—will also allow for Curcumin's health benefits in the body. Quercetin is a flavonoid (phytonutrient) that also has powerful anti-oxidant and anti-inflammatory effects which help fight against inflammation, supports respiratory and cardiovascular health, helps balance blood pressure, protects against stress and also aids in nutritional support, especially when consumed in close proximity of timeframe with Turmeric. Quercetin rich foods include: Apples, Blueberries, Cranberries, Raw Kale, Black Plums, Raw Broccoli, Red Leaf Lettuce, Red Onions, Spinach, Sweet Peppers, Chicory Greens, Snap Peas, Capers, Green Tea, Red Grapes and Red Wine.

• **S**pinach—yes, mentioning spinach again because it is loaded with vitamin E, Omega-3 fatty acids, anti-inflammatory compounds and is also high in B vitamins.

• **Chai S**eeds—contain a type of Omega-3 fatty acid called alpha-linolenic acid which also has anti-inflammatory benefits and is easily added to smoothies. yogurts, cereal, and anything you can think of.

• **G**inger—is another great anti-oxidant and anti-inflammatory that helps relieve stiffness and pain as it quickens muscle recovery.

• **S**weet **P**otatoes—are rich in beta-carotene (used by the body to make vitamin A), and are also a good source of vitamin C. Because sweet potatoes are high in anti-oxidants, such as beta-carotene and vitamin C, they offer anti-inflammatory benefits to the body. This is good news for arthritis suffers, including osteoarthritis as they may even help prevent it.

• **B**lueberries—those cute sweet little berries are easily added to yogurts and smoothies as well as fantastic on their own. They are not only anti-oxidant and anti-inflammatory, they are considered a superfood and helps with cognitive and motor function as well as combat intestinal issues and treats diarrhea with the tannins contained in them. Moderation is the key as they contain fiber.

• **S**trawberries, **B**lackberries, and **R**aspberries—Along with blueberries, these wonderfully and delightful tasting berries are power packed with antioxidants, which means they help combat inflammation, enough so that they can lower your inflammatory markers. Plus, they taste great in you know what—melted chocolate! YES! They contain tons of fiber despite their fragile little size, along with vitamins and minerals. They will boost your immunity as they lower inflammation. No wonder why my levels fluctuate (inflammatory markers) and have the doctors stumped. Hmmmm—can it be all the chocolate and strawberries I eat? I can't say for sure, but for scientific purposes, I guess I will continue to enjoy my chocolate covered strawberries!

•   **A**pples, **P**apaya & **P**ineapple—here that phytonutrient Quercetin comes into play again by aiding in recovery and reducing inflammation. Apples in particular, have higher amounts of antioxidants among fruits with their peels having a stronger source of antioxidants than the flesh. Apples are full of fiber (pectin) which additionally lowers cholesterol and inhibits cancer growth. Apples are known to reduce pain and inflammation while being protective against muscle damage. Apples also contain an important trace element, Boron, which is beneficial for bone health, enhanced brain function and immune response while reducing arthritic pain.

Papaya has many vitamins and minerals plus an inflammation and pain reducing enzyme called

Papain. This proteolytic enzyme is known to be just as effective as over the counter NSAIDS (non-steroidal anti-inflammatory drugs). Additionally, papayas contain several anti-oxidants that exhibit effects that are antihyperglycemic, antihypertensive, and anti-microbial.

Pineapple is a natural anti-inflammatory due to its vitamin C content as well as Bromelain, a protein digesting enzyme, helping with digestion, swelling and bruising as well as pain management. Pineapples are perfect for your "itis" of many forms including arthritis, tendonitis and bursitis.

• Avocados—truly are a superfood and yummy as well as versatile too. Avocados are packed with antioxidants, fiber, magnesium, potassium, vitamins, minerals, and are a healthy fat that is heart healthy. Avocados have beneficial health benefits of lowering inflammation as it increases your body's ability to absorb other nutrients and antioxidants from other plant sources. Just by adding an avocado to your salad enhances the nutritional content dramatically by increasing absorption. Plus, it adds that wonderful flavor as well as texture component.

Avocados are also beneficial in both preventing certain cancers as well as inhibiting the growth of cancerous cells in prostate cancer and reducing the negative effects of chemotherapy on lymphocytes. Note—chemotherapy is not always the way to go (it is destructive to the body, tissues, and healthy cells) as there is more success through holistic medicine via a naturopath, offering the body a chance to protect itself from cancer ever returning.

- **S**chisandra **B**erry—is great to help fight against that awful fatigue! Yeah, you know exactly what I'm talking about. This works amazingly! Not only is Schisandra Berry great for battling fatigue but also stress and depression. It is powerful in increasing endurance and stamina; just what we need. Yay!

Schisandra is also beneficial for the liver as it aids in healing and promotes proper liver function. (Don't forget the liver has a big job in filtering the blood and detoxifying chemical compounds as it also metabolizes medications and synthesizes non-essential amino acids.) That is a lot of work to do! Schisandra helps to restore by cleansing the liver after all that hard work. Not only so, it also helps boost cognitive function and benefits the brain in terms of memory as well.

Other beneficial benefits of Schisandra Berry include relieving anxiety, and helps combat adrenal fatigue, exhaustion, insomnia, dizziness, headaches, palpitation and sweating by offering relief through correcting the symptoms of adrenal fatigue and supporting healthy adrenal function and hormonal health. Schisandra is even capable of helping with bone healing and useful in preventing such diseases as osteoporosis.

Additionally, because Schisandra Berry helps combat stress it also benefits the immune system that is easily affected by stress. Its overall calming effect, along with mental alertness ability allows for normalization of blood pressure, reducing restless leg syndrome, benefits ADHD all while aiding in mental performance. Due to its anti-inflammatory properties Schisandra Berry is perfect for arthritis sufferers, chronic fatigue and Fibromyalgia. Schisandra Berry comes in capsule, powder and tincture form for a variety of ways to add to your dietary supplementation.

• Frankincense (Boswellia)—is an anti-inflammatory that binds to enzymes that cause inflammation, therefore reduces inflammation and is perfect for auto-immune support and also treats inflammatory conditions such as arthritis and Crohn's disease while it eases pain.

Frankincense is an essential oil extracted from the Boswellia Tree and is considered to be the "king" of essential oils; no wonder the three kings (wise men) gave it as a gift to the "King". Besides its anti-inflammatory benefits, Frankincense is also beneficial in helping the liver and kidneys remove toxins, aids in absorption of nutrients, strengthens the immune system, benefits digestive, respiratory and nerve health as well as the excretory and limbic systems.

Frankincense helps promote healthy cell regeneration keeping existing cells healthy. It is used to treat dry skin, minimalize scars and stretch mark appearances as well as has astringent and anti-bacterial properties and aids in wound healing. Frankincense is so beneficial to the brain/body connection and is beneficial for the hypothalamus, pituitary and pineal glands. Frankincense additionally supports memory, emotional responses and behavior as it relieves stress and anxiety. It truly is the king of essential oils. As with all essential oils, Frankincense should be diluted with a carrier oil such as coconut or mixed in water. It does however thin blood so anyone with a history of a bleeding disorder should use caution.

• **Fermented Foods/Probiotic Foods** as discussed earlier such as **K**efir has B-vitamins, biotin, enzymes, probiotics, calcium, boosts immunity, heals irritable bowel, kills candida (fungal infection in gut), and builds bone density.

Kombucha—contains B-vitamins, enzymes and probiotics, detoxes the body, improves digestion, increases energy, supports the immune system and reduces joint pain offering arthritic relief. Kombucha helps develop a stronger immunity with its anti-inflammatory and antimicrobial properties. The antioxidants and polyphenols in Kombucha help protect gastric tissue, helping to prevent and treat gastric ulcers. Kombucha additionally helps the body break down complex carbohydrates and protein, which aids in nutrient absorption and preventing toxins from being absorbed.

Probiotic **Y**ogurt— (higher protein less sugar) improves a healthier metabolic profile, blood pressure and triglyceride levels. It is best made organically from grass-fed goat or sheep. Food for thought: All those antibiotics that are pumped into cows, transfers into what we ingest from them, then has a negative effect and a big negative impact on our bodies and our health.

Pickles and **S**auerkraut— are other familiar choices of fermented foods, but not as readily eaten by most. Sauerkraut is fermented cabbage with many vitamins and minerals, beneficial in boosting digestive health as it also aids in circulation, reducing cholesterol levels, improving bone health and the big one—fights and reduces inflammation. Sauerkraut however is an acquired taste and not everyone is fond of it. Try it and decide for yourself, as the benefits will out-way the sound of its name.

Pickles, on the other hand, more people seem to be familiar with and more readily agreeable to add to their diet. Pickles, believe it or not, have plenty of vitamins and minerals—Huh, who would have thought. They also contain gut-friendly bacteria (the good kind) and also antioxidants. We are hearing that word a lot, aren't we? Pickles can even help with a vitamin K deficiency. Look for organic when choosing your picked cucumber.

There are other fermented foods less heard of, which you can research on your own, but they are very important to a healthy diet and overall homeostasis—a body in balance. They create a protective lining in the intestines and protect against pathogens (germs/bad bacteria) with the microflora that increases good intestinal flora (good bacteria). Fermented foods help build a stronger immune system by increasing antibodies as they regulate appetite and reduce cravings for sugar and refined carbs.

• **A**shwagandha— Ashwagandha is an adaptogenic herb that modulates (regulates) thyroid function, offers anti-inflammatory properties, is a neuroprotective, and acts as an anti-anxiety and anti-depressant. It supports and strengthens the immune system and acts as a protective agent against stress, helpful in lowering cortisol levels and balancing the hormones that so often go out-of-wack due to stresses and injury; such as a Traumatic Brain Injury.

Ashwagandha supports many bodily systems including endocrine, immune, neurological and even reproductive; which is very supportive when our reproductive hormones are imbalanced due to damage to the hypothalamus and pituitary gland, resulting in adrenal fatigue. Ashwagandha is known for regulating those key reproductive hormones, such as estrogen, prolactin, also DHEA and progesterone, relieving adrenal fatigue and supporting healthy sleep.

Ashwagandha additionally offers therapeutic benefits of regulating normal blood sugar levels, helping to combat Diabetes, and also increases endurance, muscle strength and stamina, improves memory and cognitive function, while reducing brain cell degeneration as it protects the brain from neurodegenerative diseases such as Parkinson's and Alzheimer's.

• **Eleuthero Root (Siberian Ginseng)**— grows as a thorny shrub, native to regions of

Siberia and Eastern Asia. It is an adaptogen that helps the body adapt to both internal and external stressors. Eleuthero root is known for enhancing physical and mental performance as well as boosts the immune system and reduces symptoms of fatigue and also reduces lactic acid formation further reducing and delaying muscle fatigue.

Note Since Eleuthero boosts the immune system, it is Not meant for auto-immune disorders because the immune system is already overactive, but it can be helpful in Chronic Fatigue Syndrome or fatigue caused by Post-Concussion Syndrome. Fibromyalgia is not currently classified as an auto-immune disease, however, since often times it does accompany auto-immune disorders, check with your health care provider before taking. ***

Eleuthero is able to assist in halting cognitive decline while improving cognitive abilities, having a regulatory effect on norepinephrine and dopamine levels in the brain, enough to delay the onset of Parkinson's disease. Eleuthero is also considered a natural mood stabilizer, reducing stress and anxiety, as it also improves memory and overall cognitive function, sharpening cognitive abilities. Other benefits of Eleuthero are known to aid in insomnia, anti-aging and detoxification.

Eleuthero is considered an antioxidant, helpful in the prevention of free-radical formation, making it effective in the prevention of cancers and offering the body many health benefits and another way to get an antioxidant in.

• **Cocao Nibs**—offer that superfood energy boost that helps battle fatigue as its antioxidant power contains more antioxidant activity than wine, tea, blueberries and even goji berries. Wow! They are so versatile that they can be added to smoothies of your choice, adding in a delicious health boost to your palate and diet. It is the flavonoids and phytonutrients in cocao nibs that give it its superpower as a supreme superfood.

The benefits of cocao nibs include improved nerve and muscle function, including keeping the heart muscle rhythm steady while enhancing nerve function. Additionally, cocao nibs help reduce the risk of coronary heart disease—beneficial in vascular and platelet function, insulin resistance, and regulating blood pressure, preventing stroke, preventing anemia, enhances mood which reduces stress levels as it acts on neurotransmitters in the brain, and also contains a high fiber content which helps you feel fuller to lose unwanted weight, as it also aids in both treating constipation and diarrhea.

- **Bone Broth**—is so remarkable to health that it truly does restore one's health. Grandma was right all along—whenever there is an ill, soup to the rescue; and for good reason! Bone broth is actually considered the #1 thing (food) to consume. Bone broth treats leaky gut, helps you to overcome allergies and food intolerances (you know that gluten that causes so many inflammatory problems that seem to last), reduces cellulite (hello-YAY), boosts the immune system, and therefore improves joint health.

Foods that offer joint health are always wonderful news, especially if anyone has ever told you that you walk like the Penguin from Batman, thinking they are being funny, as we waddle across the floor and turn with that iconic Penguin style that has our family in hysterics. We respond with, "Really?!" Yeah, I know, double quotation marks which is normally a no-no, but in this case, it fits! For curious minds longing to know if this really happened, or still does, the answer is, yes! My husband frequently meets me with that greeting. I don't know, maybe he's been watching too much Gotham. At first, I cried, but now, I can see the humor in it and laugh at it as well. It does lead me to wonder if the Penguin has an auto-immune disorder or Fibromyalgia. Hmmm...So with this humorous moment so generously offered by my husband, I let him know that this is going in the book.

Okay, back to the bone broth. Soup, chicken especially, really is good for the soul, as is beef, lamb and more. However, to receive the full healing benefits of chicken bone broth, you need to boil the parts we normally do not use, meaning the neck and feet. "What?" Yes, the chicken feet too! It becomes so incredibly nutrient dense and easily digestible.

What is boiled down is the bones and marrow, the skin, feet, tendons, ligaments, and is simmered over a period of time from at least all day (10 hours or so) to several days. What develops is a soup (broth) filled with a supply of many minerals that also contain chondroitin and glucosamine which is perfect for joint pain and far cheaper and better for you than any supplement purchased. Bone broth also contains amino acids, collagen, gelatin and trace minerals, which are smaller than macro minerals when most people talk about minerals. This will not only reduce inflammation tremendously but also reduce arthritic pain. As an added benefit our immune system is highly boosted as our gut is healed.

Bone broth protects the joints, helps us to maintain healthy skin, boosts detoxification, aids in metabolism (by playing a role in antioxidant defense with nutrient metabolism and regulation on a cellular level), enhances and helps the gut to not only repair but also restore by promoting a flourishing of healthy growth of probiotics (good bacteria).

Bone broth also helps build and repair muscle and bone density as well as improves connective tissue health. Now with many auto-immune disorders, there is considered Mixed Connective Tissue Disease when doctors cannot pinpoint which auto-immune disorder someone may be suffering from as symptoms overlap between different diseases. Bone broth can certainly help in this regard. No wonder our ancestors frequently made bone broth and did not waste any part of the animal. Bone broth is so simple, yet so amazing in its health benefits and healing. We just have to get over the idea of boiling/simmering chicken feet.

Isn't is just the most amazing and coolest thing to know that God made all these wonderful foods and herbs to help us prosper and be in good health? It truly is amazing!

Pleasant words are a honeycomb, Sweet to the soul and healing to the bones.
Proverbs 16:24 NASB

Taste and see that the LORD is good; blessed
is the one who takes refuge in him.
Psalm 34:8 NIV

What? know ye not that your body is the
temple of the Holy Ghost *which is* in you, which
ye have of God, and ye are not your own?
1 Corinthians 6:19 KJV

But whoever drinks of the water that I will give
him shall never thirst; but the water that I will
give him will become in him a well of water
springing up to eternal life."
John 4:14 NASB

Pain Relief

Normally, pain is the body's way of letting us know that something is wrong, something is dangerous, as it is a protective mechanism meant to protect us, much like an immune system normally works to protect us from enemy attacks of germs, viruses, bacteria, et cetera. If we touch something too hot, our body will send us a signal of pain through the nerves, in a sensory nervous system's response stimulation of sensory nerve cells (nociception), sending the signal along the nerve fibers in the spinal cord, up to the brain, to protect us from injury. But what happens when pain arises out of no apparent reason, without the cause being by any touch sensation whatsoever? This type of pain is characterized as being musculoskeletal in origin that is mostly caused by injury to connective tissue, muscles, tendons, ligaments, joints, bones and also to nerves.

When there is damage to nerves and nerve cells, the perception, of sensations, is altered and pain can be felt that comes from the spinal cord and brain (central nervous system); not by actual touch as in the peripheral nervous system. The amplified pain is due to disturbances in how the brain processes pain signals as well as other sensory information it receives. This helps explain the often "unexplainable" pain of Fibromyalgia pains (needle-like, shard-like, sliver-like, burning-like, that starts, stops and continues unexplainably, yet undeniably very much felt by the sufferer. These pains can happen anywhere, even visceral, in the body because the pain pathways are all amplified. Musculoskeletal pain is not just concerning Fibromyalgia as it also affects connective tissue, to additionally include Rheumatoid Arthritis and Osteoarthritis as well as tendonitis and Carpal Tunnel Syndrome.

The stiffness felt, the aching joints and muscles, the sharper pains, recurrent pains and also swelling of the joints can make mobility challenging and daunting for someone continually dealing with one form of pain or another; usually several and ongoing. Relief is not only needed in order to function properly for our activities of daily living, but it is also very much longed for; because "pain" is draining and very much exhausting. Add the tiredness of pain to the never-ending fatigue and we have a recipe for a diminished will to keep going forward joyfully, because it can be depressing.

Sometimes, all we need is a little relief, and a little hope for that sparkle of just knowing we can get through each day, every day. Natural ways of relieving pain offer a chance for the body to heal and oftentimes correct issues going on, while we get that much needed relief and comfort physically. If something is non-reversible, still natural ways offer the body the best fighting chance without causing a wave of new health concerns.

Naturally

Okay here it is! It is what most of us are waiting for, answers in pain relief "naturally" without all these crazy drugs being prescribed like candy that have negative effects on both bodily systems and the brain. Not only do some of these drugs cause issues like the dreaded constipation that no one likes to admit, but some go as far as suppressing our immune system. Let me hear you say now, "Ah, no! I like to have a functioning immune system to protect my body, thank you very much!"

Natural does come in various forms, especially if we were still talking about food. Like for instance the coined term, "natural flavoring" is natural alright. But, you may not want to eat it if you knew what it was. Okay, I will tell you. You must be dying to know. Natural flavor, in terms of vanilla sounds very nice; doesn't it? I mean, we think of vanilla beans, the pleasant smell, the delightful taste on our tongue. However, have you priced real vanilla bean? They are quite expensive. Probably too expensive for companies to add into their food "products" if they are keeping the prices of their products low.

Although sometimes natural vanilla flavoring can come from other food sources such as corn, clove or rice bran, even tree bark, it is manipulated in a lab with chemical concoctions of solvents, preservatives and other chemicals added in, to make you think you are ingesting vanilla. Apparently, we cannot tell the difference. Note: If a product does contain vanilla bean, it will say so on the label of ingredients. So, the answer to the burning question of, "What the heck is natural vanilla flavoring?" Are you ready? You might want to sit down for this answer. Food scientists are not only able to create vanilla flavor, they are also able to help companies in their plight of wanting to sell products with natural vanilla flavor at a reasonable cost. This vanilla flavor, natural don't forget, is derived from the anal glands of beavers, in their secretions. I heard that "Eww!" sound you just made. I know, Eww! Double eww and triple eww! Now that's disgusting! So, the next time you say "Yum" or "Mmmmmmm" to that natural vanilla flavor, you may quiver a bit. Not to disgust you any further, I mean, you had a brain injury. How much more can you take? However, the technical term for this pleasant/unpleasant beaver anal secretion is called, castoreum, and though it is a thick brown goo, it is said to have a pleasant smell. Sorry. You may find less food products containing this "natural" ingredient today as time goes on and people catch on, but it is also used in fragrances of perfumes and lotions as well as candle wax.

So, why am I telling you this? I'm sure you're wondering. It is to get you to be a smart consumer, to read labels and to have understanding of what it is that we put into our bodies in the name of food and also medicine. Sharing this with you as well as urging you to read both food and medicine (drug) labels pertaining not only to ingredients but also side effects, prompts you to engage your brain and exercise your thinking skills and thought processes, engaging the neurons to fire and become active as we learn. What better way to learn something new then to learn about health and how it is affected by what we put into our bodies and what may cause side effects, impair our health further or just offer an altered state of being.

We will find for instance that just because sugar cane grows, does not mean that sugar is good for you, as it feeds cancer cells as well as also relates to causing cells to mutate in the first place. Sugar also negatively affects inflammation in the body as well as causes it, in addition to a host of other health issues and diseases such as obesity and diabetes. There is enough in our processed food sources today, so if we feel the need to add more, really it should be done in moderation.

On that note, also, just because cocaine is derived from cocoa leaves naturally grown, but made into a powder, does not mean it is good for you. Additionally, just because poppy seeds are grown and come from a beautiful flowering plant, certainly does not mean that the narcotics derived from it such as opium, heroin, morphine and even codeine, made from the unripe seed capsule giving its narcotic power, is good for you either. Sure, during extreme painful situations analgesics are prescribed to help deal with excruciating pain but the addictive makeup of the drugs is causing an epidemic in our society as they are also taken recreationally, causing a plethora of problems. The non-narcotic ripe seed however is used with a culinary purpose for adding flavoring, seasoning and oil to many creative dishes.

The main thing to remember is that medication has its place and time as to when it is truly needed. But, when the side-effects out-way the benefits, it's time to look into other natural means; since we are on the topic of natural.

So often, all too often actually, drugs such as Biologics, DMARDS, and steroids are prescribed for pain resulting from inflammation, such as in cases of arthritic pain, whether they be an auto-immune disease or degenerative. Steroids as in corticosteroids, are used to lessen swelling and dampen an over active immune system. Anabolic steroids are prescribed for muscle wasting, such as with AIDS patients under medical supervision. Athletes will sometimes destructively use anabolic steroids, to build extreme muscle, that are a synthetic version of testosterone, hurting their bodies in the process; though testosterone that is naturally produced by both men and woman in the human body is helpful, as are other hormones. Synthetic anabolic steroids are very powerful and can cause a host of serious health risks including tendon rupture, heart attacks and cancer, to name only a few. Synthetic versions of any hormone come with added health risks.

Corticosteroids although are given to treat such auto-immune conditions such as Lupus, Rheumatoid Arthritis, Gout, Sjogren's syndrome, rashes, asthma, et cetera, to treat inflammation, come with great concern for their side-effects which include acne, muscle weakness, insomnia, increased body hair, weight gain, blurred vision and cataracts as well as glaucoma, easy bruising, high blood pressure, mood and memory problems, thinning bones (causing risk for fractures), also lowers the resistance to infection (placing a person at risk for infections) and further suppresses adrenal gland hormone production. Doesn't this sound like a crazy loop in how we got here in the first place?

The disconnect between the brain and body happened, between the brain and the adrenal glands, between the brain and the gut, and the interruption of communication from severed and damaged neurons and stretched axons. Communication was all scrambled. Diet and environment added to the upheaval. So now, we are supposed to just take some drugs that will enhance and disrupt us further by only masking the symptoms? Say it isn't so! That ultimately places a person at risk for infections and further health problems. In this case, the risks out-way the benefits, especially since there are so many natural ways in dealing with pain, swelling and stiffness.

Biologics are drugs that are designed to help reduce inflammation with the idea to minimalize joint damage through targeting certain proteins and cells, such as "T cells", your immune system's natural killer cells meant to protect you from pathogens and "B Cells" that produce antibodies to fight against pathogenic antigens as well as mature into memory B cells to remember the antigen (foreign pathogen), to protect you further. Biologics work by suppressing the immune system, the same immune system that you were born with to keep you healthy by fighting off the armies of germs, viruses, and bacteria that we come in contact with on a daily basis. We then put ourselves at risk for serious infections. If we only think we're sick now, just wait. If we decide to take a biologic drug, which is manufactured from living organism's cells and proteins by recombinant DNA technology (cloning), we may be in for very unpleasant times. Biologics are usually given when disease modifying antirheumatic drugs (DMARDS) have not worked. Risks can include fungal infections, tuberculosis, chest pain, difficulty breathing, change in blood pressure, dizziness, rash, flu-like symptoms, headaches, cough, abdominal discomfort and many more. These are far too many unnecessary and unwelcomed symptoms, as well as life threatening.

So now, this same immune system that was designed to protect us will be suppressed, inactive in a sense to fight for us. Although, something went haywire with it to cause it to become "overactive", as in the case of an auto-immune disease, it suddenly lies dormant. But, then what happens? Here comes along an attack from an outside source and our main defenses are down. We had better not go anywhere other than live in a bubble. But, I am not ready to become "bubble girl"! Are you ready to become "bubble boy" or "bubble girl"? Heck no! I would be screaming "Let me out!"

Most doctors seem to be becoming on board to the healthy natural alternative ways to treat inflammation and auto-immune disorders, other than most Rheumatologists that is. Why? Guess it's their job. Just like a surgeon cuts open, removes or fixes then sews up, and most doctors prescribe pharmaceutical drugs for each symptom, missing the big picture as a whole, in what the underlying cause really is, and a Pharmacist fills the prescriptions prescribed, just as a "Rheumy" (Rheumatologist) tries to stop the inflammation with drugs—maybe just so we stop complaining.

But, we're not complaining per se, we just want to know the facts. We want to know what we actually have going on in our bodies and how to stop it with minimal risk. If it is easy as naturally changing our diets, ingesting gut healing and protecting foods, brain boosting foods that also help in our daily functioning, and exercise that will help with all those necessary brain/body connections, then, why aren't we? That is a huge question. It does not take a degree nor is it rocket science to understand that if we do what's best and give what's best to our human bodies, then our body will respond by taking care of us. Our body is quite capable of healing. We see that every time we get a boo-boo, a minor injury like a cut. Our body heals itself. We are made that way to have a self-healing mechanism going on within our bodies.

Other natural means for the sake of health benefits would include plants, roots and herbs that are beneficial to the human body and does indeed help with inflammation and pain as some offer natural anti-inflammatories, antioxidants, amino acids as well as antibiotic, antifungal and antiviral properties without the side-effects so commonly found within medications. A list of such beneficial plants are as follows.

• **Moringa Oleifera:** Moringa is a highly nutritious superfood with powerful anti-inflammatory, antioxidant and protective properties that are perfect for relieving arthritic pain as it is naturally anti-inflammatory.

Moringa is additionally helpful in the battle of arthritic swelling, tenderness, stiffness in addition to pain relief with its strong analgesic and anti-inflammatory properties as it suppresses the inflammation that causes pain, as well as reduces pain, making it very beneficial and helpful in auto-immune disorders such as Rheumatoid Arthritis, Osteoarthritis and others as well as being effective in Fibromyalgia pain felt within the joints, tender points and throughout the widespread pain in the body. Moringa can additional reduce heart risks that can accompany many arthritic conditions including auto-immune disorders where the body attacks organs such as the heart.

• **Turmeric:** Turmeric is a proven natural pain killer that is also an effective natural anti-inflammatory, more so than NSAIDS (over the counter non-steroidal anti-inflammatory drugs). Turmeric is said to out-perform common arthritic drugs; it is that effective!

Turmeric also helps with neuropathy related pain as it inhibits the production of proteins responsible for expressing the pain. The curcumin in Turmeric helps intervene the pain receptors (pain arising from stimulation of the nerve cells—nociceptive), halting the pain. Turmeric additionally reduces depression symptoms that often accompany chronic pain and even boosts skin health with its antioxidant properties. Turmeric is also being widely used with success in both treating and preventing cancers; all without the harsh side-effects that accompany traditional cancer treatments.

• **Frankincense Essential Oil (Boswellia):** Frankincense is commonly grown in Somalia and is made from the resin of the Boswellia Carterii or the Boswellia Sacra Tree. It offers strong anti-inflammatory properties as well as others anti-cancer benefits in addition to boosting immunity. Frankincense works through the Limbic System in the brain, influencing the nervous system, relieving pain.

Frankincense also helps reduce anxiety, stress and depression that so often accompanies pain, especially chronic pain. Its immune enhancing abilities help destroy bacteria, viruses, even cancers and also has antiseptic qualities. Cognitively, Frankincense helps improve memory both short and long-term as well as improves learning abilities. Frankincense additionally helps fight fatigue and balances hormonal levels.

For pain management and reduction, Frankincense inhibits the production of key inflammatory molecules that cause so much pain and further prevents the breakdown of cartilage tissues, making it a great benefit for arthritis sufferers or anyone suffering from joint, muscle or tendon pain.

• **Arnica Montana:** Arnica is well known and frequently prescribed by doctors practicing the benefits of natural healing for its anti-inflammatory, analgesic and antiseptic properties as well as reduction in bruising after surgical procedures. Arnica is a perennial herb native to Europe and North America that is used topically as a cream or gel, as well as orally under the tongue in tiny dissolvable pill form. Arnica is used for pain management after surgeries, trauma and even for diabetic retinopathy (a complication of diabetes effecting the vision—floaters, distortions, blurred visions and microaneurysms).

When using arnica for pain, there is reported decreases in pain along with decreases in bruising and quicker healing times for injuries. Arnica is beneficial for treating arthritis and may be even more effective than non-steroidal anti-inflammatory drugs such as ibuprofen. Arnica gel can be applied directly over joints in the hands for pain, three times a day, with reported effective pain relief along with improved hand function. Since Arnica can be taken in a variety of ways, its ease and effectiveness are perfect for muscles and joints having inflammation, offering needed relief.

• **Tart Cherry Juice:** Tart Cherry juice, rich in potassium and iron is sour to the taste but provides higher amounts of anthocyanins (pigments and flavonoids with the ability to protect the body against disease), promoting anti-inflammatory processes within the body. Because tart cherry juice contains so much antioxidant value, it is perfect for pain relief as it fights inflammation and reduces swelling that causes pain. It also regulates metabolism as it fights abdominal fat. The rich potassium levels in tart cherry juice are beneficial for the electrical nerve impulses, heart rate, muscle recovery from exercising, blood pressure, hydration and also regulating the pH balance within the body. It offers a positive impact on the immune system with its infection fighting abilities through the high antioxidant, anti-viral and also anti-cancer properties.

• **SAMe**: SAMe is short for S-adenosylmethionine, that is effective pain relief for arthritis, joint health and mobility, healthy liver function, mood and emotional well-being, and even Fibromyalgia through a process called methylation, (the passing exchange of chains of molecules in the body),

SAMe being the ultimate donor to the methyl group for everything to run smoothly. SAMe acts as the "stick" in the relay race of life, for the runners to keep running the race. SAMe donates this methyl group whenever needed by the body; lack of it turns everything sluggish with experiences of lack of energy along with impaired functions.

When there is impaired methylation, there is also impaired brain and bodily functions as it benefits both brain and joint activity; therefore, SAMe is a perfect treatment for depression, arthritis, as well as a liver tonic. ***SAMe however should not be used for depression with bipolar disorders unless under medical supervision due to the possibility of worse bipolar episodes.

As for pain management, SAMe is said to reduce pain by at least 20% in clinical trials, which is the same effectiveness as nonsteroidal anti-inflammatories such as ibuprofen. SAMe possesses anti-inflammatory, pain relieving and tissue healing properties that may even help protect the joints, as well as reduce tender points on the body with regards to Fibromyalgia.

• **Evening Primrose Oil:** Evening Primrose Oil has been known to help restore nerve function in peripheral neuropathy and also help relieve the pain associated by providing gamma-linolenic acid (omega-6 fatty acid); beneficial in fighting chronic inflammation. The "GLA" in Evening Primrose Oil works by preventing additional damage to nerve cells, inhibiting myelin degeneration, protecting axon length, correcting nerve conduction, assisting in nerve repair while regulating the inflammatory process; restoring proper nerve function and helpful in Fibromyalgia.

•   **CBD** oil: Cannabidiol (CBD) for short, is a chemical compound made from cannabis, but it is not psychoactive like marijuana is. CBD acts against the THC, (tetrahydrocannabinol), one of the 113 cannabinoids in cannabis, targeted receptors to reduce the negative effects such as anxiety and paranoia that often accompanies inhaling or ingesting weed. CBD oil (for pain relief) is thought to bind to the serotonin receptors while reducing inflammation and alleviating pain.

As CBD reduces the psychoactive symptoms, it eases mood by positively affecting it and reduces anxiety, calming mental function, being a mood regulator. It is used also to lower blood pressure in people suffering from high blood pressure. CBD is used successfully in cancer patients, much like medical marijuana for pain. CBD mostly interacts throughout the brain/body via the endocannabinoid system (receptors in skin, bone, organs, central nervous system, etc.) via neurotransmitters that bind to cannabinoid receptors and cannabinoid receptor proteins throughout the central nervous system and peripheral nervous system, attempting to regulate memory, mood, cognitive processes, pain sensations and appetite. It acts in a sense along the lines of an endocannabinoid (the neurotransmitter anandamide) that increases during physical activity such as running, giving that sense of a "runners high". CBD oil offers the positives effects without the psychotropic high and associated paranoia.

It is important to monitor overall improvement in health with regard to mood, sleep, and pain levels and alleviation of symptoms for optimal dosage and therapeutic results. It is also important to note that it should continually be in your system for better results. Look for CBD oil that is third party tested for contaminants as well as active ingredients (free of contaminants where grown and processed), extracted from therapeutic cannabinoid rich hemp and manufactured in a registered lab that follows GMP (good manufacturing practices) standards and AHPA (American Herbal Products Association) guidelines. Happy Hemping!

- **M**edical or **L**egal **M**arijuana (**C**annabis) per your region: This seems to be the next obvious inquiry when it comes to pain management, but the decision is completely your own. You will need to weigh out the pro's and con's. A pro (benefit) would be that it does have therapeutic benefits and does work for pain relief. A con would be that you will be under a psychotropic and negative influence (if with THC) which could alter your sense of being in that you may not be of sound mind, which could make you susceptible in the spirit realm for being influenced out of your control, giving you feelings of anxiety, panic attacks, noticeable mood swings, and even paranoia.

> ***What also can be noticed is a rapid heart rate (tachycardia), low blood pressure (hypotension)—therefore may also experience dizziness and lightheadedness, in addition to impaired motor skills, decreased gastrointestinal motility, and muscle relaxation.

The negative emotional feelings of paranoia can start suddenly and most abruptly, even in the middle of an otherwise euphoric relaxed or heightened mood. If this makes no sense to you, skip to the next. However, if this does make some sense or ring a bell (just not your bell—we don't want any more brain injuries), or even if you want to learn more, educate yourself on spiritual warfare as it definitely does exist. Just be cautious if choosing to use this and don't give into any abnormal behaviors or choices other than what you would normally do without being under any influence.

Other medicinal uses of cannabis that have been beneficial is in the use of treating cancer patients and off-setting the terrible side-effects of chemotherapy drugs, helping to reduce nausea and vomiting, relieve anxiety, while promoting better sleep and appetite. It is already widely used to treat ailments of sleep apnea, hypertension, osteoporosis, Alzheimer's, HIV/AIDS, MS (Multiple Sclerosis), ALS (Lou-Gehrig's Disease), and Fibromyalgia.

If you are already quite privy to pot/weed and don't have a problem with anything disturbing, then I would recommend eating it or via sublingual tincture, rather than smoking it (if it is legal in your state or region—you don't want to get in trouble now), and also rather than vaporizing or using inhalers due to lung involvement. You don't want to have a lung problem on top of everything else, especially smoking it will definitely be inflammatory to your lungs, damage cells and put you at risk for lung cancer. Since the THC in marijuana is fat soluble (stored in the body's fat tissues slowly entering the blood stream), and most effective when consumed with fat, adding it to butter or coconut oil is best, and is also complimentary with chocolate. Ingesting it which includes via oils, liquids and capsules is better for everyone.

Plus, if it's legal in your area, do you really want to get everyone else high around you too—the kids, cats, dogs, birds? That would be bad and could be life-threatening for them. Just make sure it's in a safe place for your pain relief.

The decision to use medical/legal marijuana (cannabis) is a decision that only you can make along with your health care provider.

• ***I cover the horrifying risks of taking Gabapentin for pain relief in the Fibromyalgia chapter and advise against it. Please refer to that chapter and also educate yourself further on the risks and drug interactions with other drugs that depress the CNS; which only further increases the risks.***

• **Ganoderma (Reishi Mushroom)**— Ganoderma, is a mushroom supplement I've discussed earlier in the diet section for its wide array of health benefits and is available as a supplement in either dried (powdered), capsule or extract/tincture form. It is also available in a coffee blend (see back of book for info. under "important links"). Ganoderma is naturally antibacterial, antifungal and antiviral with the ability to lower inflammation and improve blood circulation which helps to resolve infections, reduce pain and inflammation, aches, and stiffness as well as fight fatigue which can very often accompany pain. Since

Ganoderma is an adaptogen, regulating the immune system, it works wonderfully for pain relief as it regulates and restores normal immune function, ultimately reducing inflammation causing pain.

And said, I cried by reason of mine affliction unto the LORD, and he heard me; out of the belly of hell cried I, *and* thou heardest my voice.
Jonah 2:2 KJV

The LORD is my rock, my fortress, and my savior; my God is my rock, in whom I find protection. He is my shield, the power that saves me, and my place of safety.
Psalm 18:2 NLT

And He said, "My presence shall go with you, and I will give you rest."
Exodus 33:14 NASB

He will wipe every tear from their eyes. There will be no more death or mourning or crying or pain, for the old order of things has passed away."
Revelation 21:4 NIV

Exercise

Exercise is perfect for not only gaining and maintaining strength, but also for mobility, flexibility, endurance, emotional health, energy, recovery, and also helps repair damage in the brain. It improves the circulatory system by strengthening the heart and lowering blood pressure, in addition to helping with weight management and also controlling blood sugar levels.

When we suffer from disorders such as auto-immune diseases or Fibromyalgia, we are most often fatigued and in pain, which can dampen our physical activity posing risks for weakness, loss of muscle tone and also depression from lack of exercise, not to mention more pain and susceptibility to further injury and other disease processes. That does not have to be the case though because a low impact and aerobic (requiring oxygen to help improve our cardiovascular system) form of exercise, such as waking and swimming, can actually be beneficial in improving (disrupted) sleep, improving self-esteem, helping with pain management, and reducing stress as well as depression. Sometimes the hardest part is just starting. But, once we start and keep it up several times throughout the week, it then becomes a habit, a good and beneficial habit that we can continue to do for ourselves to feel better.

Movements of motor function, even the simplest for most people, can become a complex motor task within the brain, within the Primary Motor Cortex. Movements through the flow of different exercises as well as one's that mostly engage the brain by tracking movements of an object such as a ball, stimulate the brain's neurons to grow as it also reduces inflammation. Regular exercise can improve memory and thinking abilities, which is so longed for from a brain inured individual. Exercise stimulates the release of growth factors, chemicals that can have a positive effect on the health of brain cells, also stimulating the growth of new blood vessels within the brain, increasing the survival of new brain cells.

Exercise is also important in its role of having a positive effect on mood and improved sleep by reducing stress and anxiety. There have even been studies that show improvements in memory and cognitive thinking abilities due to a greater volume of cells in regions of the brain, for instance, in the medial temporal cortex and the prefrontal cortex, which will help with brain fog as well. With that being said, pay close attention to your body and the cues it gives you both during and after you exercise.

When first starting out, getting cleared from your doctor first is a wise choice, however keep in mind that they may clear you when you may not be fully ready, as in the case of exerting too much pressure in your head. If you are used to lifting heavy weights and generally perform exercises with your head hung lower, then there will be extra pressure to the head from increased blood flow. I would advise against heavy exercise though you may be well versed in it.

Why? You had a brain injury and you do not want a prolonged healing or a rebound effect, equivalent to a second impact. Though things may seem fine on the outside, there is still much healing going on the inside, within your brain. Just don't push your limits. When your body says, "it's enough", it is!

I personally learned the hard way after being cleared from my doctor at the time, as well as from the physical therapist, for exercise. The point is, even though you can walk briskly on a treadmill does not mean you can lift heavy weights! There is a big difference!

At first of course, when your freshly injured, you need to be able to even walk first before adding in other forms of exercise. You may find that although your legs are able to move and have applied pressure during the re-learning of mobility, in the mild exercise of walking, you may lean over to a side and even tip over as you may have imbalances and proprioception challenges to yet overcome.

So, walking at first may be a challenge. It sure was for me. At first, I needed someone to just hang onto, otherwise I would end up who knows where. You may want to do the same. Don't forget all the bombarding stimuli of sights, smells and sounds as they will all play a role in your concentration of just trying to walk in a forward motion. Additionally, terrain, well, that has its own bag of worms. Grass, gravel, stone, cement, blacktop, leaf covered ground and also the bright white snow with added depth all make for a challenging journey. Just don't get discouraged; think of it as an adventure that although you have been on before in terms of your environment and surroundings, it's suddenly all new again. Which in a way is pretty amazing, almost like living life over again by re-learning the skill of walking. As for running, get the walking down pat first. When you do, man, you will run the race with endurance. Just be cautious of the brain bouncing inside your head and monitor for any unpleasant symptoms.

Once you're good at walking again, as practice does make better, you may notice a fast pace going on which is great because then it becomes more aerobic in nature, therefore is said to boost the size of the hippocampus, which is a good thing because that area of the brain is involved in learning and verbal memory. You know all too well I'm sure, the memory problems going on. So, let's do some walking. If you can regularly exercise, say at least three to four times a week, the benefits will be astounding, not only in neuro connections and cardiovascular health but also good for your booty too.

Exercise is something we all need to maintain health, flexibility, mobility, cardiovascular health as well as emotional health, because your body releases "feel good" endorphins as your self-esteem also improves. Lack of exercise is linked to depression and depressive thoughts. People who regularly engage in some form of physical activity have a more positive mood and uplifting spirit; and if we can do it with a friend or two, it is then all the more enjoyable as we're all in it together. Now understandably, when someone undergoes a brain injury and then is diagnosed with an auto-immune disorder, there are limitations that are to be expected. With that being said, when you are ready and able, game on to try a little.

With auto-immune diseases as well as with Fibromyalgia, there is going to be stiffness and soreness of joints as our body responds to what is happening within us. There is going to be difficulty moving at times, sometimes more so than others. There are going to be times when you are sure you've come down with either "turtlenervosis" or even "snailitis" for extreme slowness in moving about, as everyone else seems to be flying by you. That is okay. Just pace yourself the best you can. Just imagine a wonderful armour on you, much like a snail and turtle have, only better! If you are a person of faith, you know what I'm talking about. If not, look into the full Armour of God and wear it daily, even if you are at a snail's pace. It is your complete protection.

Now although you may be stiff and sore, you still need to move about, so you don't freeze up in that same stagnant position. You know how when you visit a nursing home or long-term care facility and you see all these people just sitting there with there hands in a fixed clenched position, some of them with their limbs fixed as well, don't let that be you. Not yet! You need to get up and move as much as you can, and you know what? You will be able to move around and accomplish what you don't "feel" like doing, and your pain may even lessen as you do. As much as it may hurt or feel uncomfortable with your feet hurting and your knees aching, and let's not forget about the hips bothering you, as you move you are maintaining the mobility your joints need. To make it easier you can try cushier shoes and softer ground with even surfaces, (because you don't want to twist your ankle or fall into a hole)—dogs love to dig holes. Mine at home sure does.

We just can't let the fear of pain stop us. You may moan and groan, but you can do it if you are not wheelchair bound. So, bring a cane for support if you need to. No one really cares. If they do, you can just wack em'. No seriously don't do that because then you will have another issue to deal with. Okay, maybe bring a friend to hold onto instead. Two's company anyway.

Something to note regarding auto-immune diseases and Fibromyalgia, there is already ongoing stress within us as we perceive and experience any symptoms. This stress sensitizes the Limbic System that may increase discomfort because the amygdala (in the Medial Temporal Lobe) of the Limbic System processes the input from all our sensory systems—sight, smell hearing, taste, and very importantly, touch. Since the amygdala is considered the entry to the Limbic System and passes the "sensory input" onto the hypothalamus, (the hypothalamus being the control center of the Limbic System), and remember it is connected to the pituitary gland and also to the Autonomic Nervous System (displaying bodily expressions to emotional responses), when there is damage due to a brain injury, the resulting response will also be different; hence increased painful stimuli to an otherwise light touch.

Patience may surely be needed in these such cases, even when it comes to exercise. We just may not be able to do what we did before, lift what we've lifted before, or perform as pain free as we did prior to injury. We may even react tearfully in response to a sensation or attempted exercise, that may make no sense to anybody else, as they clearly do not feel our pain, because their brains have not been altered quite the same way as ours has.

It is important to note that part of the amygdala's function in the Limbic System is processing stimuli both positive and not, and also takes into account memories. (Remember that brain injury that happened? The amygdala does!) This means, if a "perceived" threat is facing a person, there could be a "fight-or-flight" response in order to react as a defense mechanism in the brain trying to protect you—even if it's not "real". It also can have some definite impact on you if you are driving or even just a passenger in a car, thinking that the other cars are too close and that you may hit. You may react in a fear response, or perhaps even anger if it was a car accident that caused your injury.

The emotional responses that we have in reaction to these perceived threats as well as the cycle of repeated discomfort that we feel, can in a way fuel itself. They become in a sense hard-wired and difficult to overcome as we try to re-train our brains in adapting to all types of stimuli. This hard-wired new set of reactions can also impact our movements as related to sensory stimuli such as touch. What helps to interrupt this cycle is biofeedback and neurofeedback, to teach the brain to self-regulate and to train voluntary control; which I will be discussing in the "tools" section. This reset will help responses to be calmer, both within the mind as well as within the body. Infrared light has even been used to help offer relief and reduce anxiety, tension and stressful responses.

So, don't be too hard on yourself when you "can't"—because someday you "can". After all, you had a brain injury, a major inflammatory process with devastating effects cascading throughout your entire body! Your entire being has been through the ringer and your brain has undergone a battle that has made you a warrior! Just keep going and don't ever, ever give up!

With just a little exercise, we can help our bodies and our brains as we start to feel better about things, while the feel-good endorphins are released and interact with receptors in our brain, reducing our perception of pain; just by us starting to move around. We will both feel better and also look better too. We can enjoy the freshness of outdoors or listen to soft music or a recording of our choice, to help pass the time as we become healthier, physically, emotionally and spiritually. We may also find that our fatigue will lessen up a bit as well. Doesn't that sound wonderful?

Once we are able to lift weights (start lighter and work our way up to heavier without causing head pressure—remembering to breathe) they will help us maintain our muscle tone. A little goes a long way. Remember, we're not ready, ever, for being all wrinkly and floppy. I know I'm not. So, pump it! Pumping it can come from not only weight lifting but also by engaging muscle groups and squeezing them as you take turns in moving your arms and legs. You can start by focusing on one muscle group at a time and flex-n-hold-release, flex-n-hold-release, flex-n-hold-release. This can be coined active range of motion exercises or "dynamic tension". You can go through an entire range of motion for each body part, doing full arm, then wrist, circles frontwards and backwards, finger flexing and extending as well as taking turns opposing your thumb against each finger, in addition to opening and closing of fists.

Legs and butt exercises can be extension (leg straight, flexion (bent knee) and squeezing muscles (both legs and butt). You may also want to try lying down on your back as you raise your legs to make circles, starting smaller then working up to larger circles while holding in your abs (tummy). This will work both your legs and your abs. Another great exercise and seemingly simple one is to do a plank. You get down on all fours on the floor, rest upon your forearms, lift up off your knees onto your toes and hold that position for one minute while holding in your abs tightly. For this you may welcome a distraction to focus on, such as reading or listening to music because this can get difficult real fast. You may never see the length of one minute quite the same way again. When you're good at that, increase the time of hold to two minutes. This will all help build muscle strength, core strength, as well as improve mobility.

Stretching exercises will help with the much desired as well as much needed flexibility. We don't want to be all contracted up and permanently stiff before our time, with a permanent shortening of muscles and joints with constriction of our connective tissues, including ligaments and skin. No, that would be awful! We may feel like a zombie in some sort of horror flick, looking for brains; perhaps because ours was impaired and damaged. We must keep as mobile as we can, for as long as we can. We need to move our bodies as much as allowed and is possible.

Stretching will also increase blood flow helping the body get the nutrients where they need to go, for instance your cartilage and muscles, also promoting organ function and cell growth. Stretching additionally helps with injury prevention. Did you know that stretching helps with stress? Now doesn't that sound wonderful? When are muscles are all tensed up from stress, they contract, which can also negatively impact our mind. We don't want any more of that. Stretching will loosen those tight muscles and help with relaxing. If we stretch before bed, we may even sleep better too. Many stores sell exercise/fitness bands to help aid in stretching.

When we stretch the back muscles, especially the lower, along with chest and shoulders we help with our posture as this creates a better alignment in our spine. Stretching will also increase our stamina, relieving muscle fatigue while loosening muscles and tendons. Although we may feel tired and even fatigued after exercising, overall when stretching is added, it will improve our energy levels by giving us a quick boost of energy, especially when we feel sluggish and quickly perform some stretching exercises. Now we know we all want more energy. It will revitalize and reinvigorate us to just keep going throughout our day.

When we exercise, especially when we are not used to doing it or when we are working on a body part we haven't worked on in a short bit, we can expect to feel some muscle soreness for having worked them. They are now in need of repair through proper nutrition and blood flow. Therefore, stretching helps to minimize the discomfort by allowing the supply of nutrients to get to those muscles by the increased blood flow. This will overall help with any athletic performance, even for beginners and those who just want to be a little more mobile. In addition, Arnica helps with muscle soreness as muscles heal and repair from exercises.

I don't mean to make light of or knock the damaging effects of immobility when I discussed being contracted up, but if it can be prevented, it should. We can't give into that, if at all possible. That being said, I also understand the devastating, debilitating and disabling effects of paralyzing diseases such as ALS (amyotrophic lateral sclerosis), MS (multiple sclerosis), Muscular Dystrophy, and Cerebral Palsy to name a few, as well as the massive need for great compassion, care, understanding, support and comfort for individuals and their families alike.

We should never judge anyone due to their outward appearance or what we can only see, because there is much more to the person on the inside and the wonderful human being that they are, we all are, and that they were created to be. They still, as we all do, at any point in life, have much to offer. Even though somebody may have a disease or disorder, they are still a gift to this world and a wonderful contribution to mankind, as are you or anybody else. Nobody wants to be sick or disabled. Nobody asked for it. We all have something in this life we would rather not have. But, we can take what we do have and still find joy in the process, even in the heat and pain of it all. Remember, nobody can steal your joy! So, don't let them.

Don't feel down with whatever your diagnosis may be. Do the best you can in the beautiful new day, each and every day, that you have been given. You are fearfully and wonderfully made. So, fight, fight to the end. Do the most for your body in order to help it, not hurt it. Don't take it for granted, ever. Don't let other things take precedence over your health and well-being and that of your family's or other relationships.

Be forever thankful for who you are and what you have as well as whatever you are dealing with, even if it is a difficult time of trial in your life. Who knows who may benefit from you and what you are going through. You may be here at this point, going through this trial and circumstance for such a time as this. Don't give up but get closer to your maker throughout both the good times as well as the bad. If these are considered the bad times for you, guess what, you're closer now than ever. You are actually at your highest when you are at your lowest! Smile! God loves you, no matter your circumstance, disability, or disease! Let Him be your strength.

He gives strength to the weary, And to him who
lacks might He increases power.
Isaiah 40:29 NASB

For physical training is of some value, but
godliness has value for all things, holding
promise for both the present life and the life to
come.
Timothy 4:8 NIV

I discipline my body like an athlete, training it
to do what it should. Otherwise, I fear that after
preaching to others I myself might be
disqualified.
1 Corinthians 9:27 NLT

She girds herself with strength And makes her arms strong.
Proverbs 31:17 NASB

Effective Tools

Tools are helpful, tools are handy, often portable and economical. Tools are essential in our therapeutic outlook for recovery. Tools are those little things that really help in big, big ways. Here are just a few handy tools that are not only useful in helping you get through your activities of daily living, they are also beneficial in the healing and recovery process, no matter how long you have been afflicted. They offer promise and hope in brain communication within our disconnected being. New connections are made within the brain, and then translates and receives information throughout our body, helping us notice real improvement along with a sense of accomplishment. They are meant to assist, engage, challenge, and allow us to go further in our recovery, since perhaps our previous therapy tools, as they also offer support. These are simple, yet very effective in what they can do.

Sanddune Stepper Rehabilitation

Such a fantastic tool that helps with the onslaught of "new challenges" relating to a Traumatic Brain Injury and Post-Concussion Syndrome is called the Sanddune Stepper. The Sanddune Stepper is a remarkable therapy tool for rehabilitation that you can utilize in your very own home at minimal cost compared to repeated doctor and physical therapy visits. Not only so, but when we start investigating neurofeedback and the much-needed benefits it has on the recovering body and brain connection, only to find out that it is not covered by most insurances, our sense of hope goes down the drain as the cost of each visit is quite expensive; too expensive especially if you have been out of work or only work very minimally due to the brain injury in the first place. It is the catch that keeps most people in the endless loop of defeat due to their current condition. But, let me bring some light into your gloom as the Sanddune Stepper can be a little life saver as it offers neurofeedback in a compact and portable form.

There has been extensive research with terrific results for those suffering from Parkinson's Disease, balance issues, proprioception challenges, as well as those in need of core stabilizing exercises and physical strength training, all while being comfortable and easy on the joints. It is absolutely perfect for TBI's (Traumatic Brain Injury) and PCS (Post-Concussion Syndrome) as it helps retrain your brain while bringing into alignment your balance as it also helps effectively re-teach your brain to know where your body is, in time and space—perfect for the proprioception challenged individual, such as myself. I really love mine and have seen such huge improvements in remarkably brief time frames.

When there are problems with one's proprioception, frequently experienced by brain injured individuals, there are challenges in how the brain receives sensory information from sensory receptors called proprioceptors that are located in the muscles, tendons, joints as well as the inner ear, that use internal stimuli to detect changes in our body's position and movement. These proprioceptors help us to detect where we are at in time and space; sensing changes in muscles to help us to keep our balance. This is accomplished by the body without the help of sight or sound. This is why, when after suffering a brain injury, a doctor will often have us stand with our arms extended outward and our eyes shut, to check if we are able to stay balanced, to stay standing upright without falling over. When our proprioception is off, we will tip over and lose our balance because there is a miscommunication of where we are at in time and space as our receptors are unable to sense changes in position and to correctly signal the central nervous system properly. An altered proprioception can also affect our hand and eye coordination when attempting to grasp objects and even perform tasks such as driving a car.

Among our proprioceptors are also interoceptors and exteroceptors. Interoceptors relate information and sensation concerning our internal environment with regard to our visceral organs, including our gut, (brain/gut connection again) relating to pain, pressure or distention. Exteroceptors connect with sights, sounds, smells and cutaneous touch sensations relaying skin sensations such as light touch, temperature, itching, tickling, pressure and superficial pain. These proprioceptors are just beneath the skin's surface in the muscles, joints, and tendons with many of the exteroceptors being on the feet sensing and attempting to relay information with every foot placement we make. Senses that are generally noticed are movements, position, vibration and also our equilibrium. When our proprioception is off, so is our equilibrium. This is why we lose balance, can become dizzy and disoriented, perceive things as closer than they are, especially when driving or riding in a car and can in addition add to the experience of fight-or-flight episodes because our brain incorrectly relates to the stimuli of mixed information.

Since there are an abundant amount of exteroceptors on our feet, more so than any other part of our body, the unique design of the Sanddune Stepper helps to correct proprioception imbalances by re-training the brain about where we are at in time and space, to more efficiently and correctly relay sensory information. The brain gathers the information relayed such as posture, position, force of each foot movement, impact, stability, and then makes appropriate changes in our muscles, tendons, and ligaments, protecting our connective tissues and joints with any adjustments necessary. The Sanddune mimics walking on sand with an absorption of force that allows for comfortable walking movements while new connections are being formed. This is why it is best to walk bare footed whenever we can, and especially on the Sanddune to help relay proper information and perform the therapeutic neurofeedback.

The Sanddune has shown clinical observations of the ability to withstand rapid movements and stepping of feet without one foot disrupting the other, therefore improving balance due to its smart design of a division between the two pads. Because of its design, a person suffering from fatigue, which is so common with an auto-immune disease, are able to improve their resistance to fatigue through rapid stepping. Rapid stepping has also helped people suffering from Parkinson's by observed improved gait on firm surfaces following just a three-minute session on the stepper; which offers hope and promise for many neurological disorders.

The Sanddune Stepper is a low impact, easy on the joints, uniquely made very thick type of memory-like foam with a high and low side containing a density that perfectly allows for a communication pathway for the Central Nervous System via neurofeedback. It is specially designed for any age as well as weight, and offers sufficient room for foot placement, pivoting and walking. It has such a sturdy base that you really feel safe as you engage your brain like never before. Its unique, one of a kind construction allows for non-compressive forces while enhancing proper co-contraction of muscles which distinctively promotes efficient movement patterns. It sends signals to your brain with every movement you make, right to the limbic system which creates a loop of neurofeedback. Essentially it re-trains your brain. It allows the body to return to relying on the feet, as you move through space and time (your immediate surroundings) as it also develops your core stabilizing system, improving balance and leg strength as well.

Once you step onto the Sanddune you will notice your center of gravity and therefore will want to maintain it throughout movements. Have something or someone close by initially until you notice significant improvements incase your center of gravity is off and you become imbalanced.

A neurofeedback loop is created by alternating fast and slow interval movements of the feet. Moving the feet at variable speeds mimics real movements in real life situations. You can also pivot the feet to the right, then to the left, for those quick motions in real life that has us changing our position at a moment's notice. At first you may notice, and actually feel that there is a connection going on within your brain that is responding to your bodily movements. The feeling may be a bit overwhelming at first, so you will want to have something sturdy to grab onto if you become initially off-balance as your body adjusts to the new movements and learning where it actually is in time and space. It will get better, quickly as your brain adapts to your body's signals. There are new connections being made at a pace that is astounding. You may soon begin to see results as your symptoms to injury or disease are becoming less bothersome and you find yourself doing more before symptoms start again. It is an effective way to boost the healing and repairing process.

The Sanddune also offers relief and help for those suffering from the effects of auto-immune diseases with much joint pain. Since it is low impact, it is perfect to get the much-needed exercise in, as well as treat the devastating effects of auto-immune diseases by lifting yourself up a bit while standing to perform a mock weightless feeling. The effects signal the brain right away as relief benefits are much welcomed.

In effectively managing auto-immune disorders, it is essential, critical even, to have a healthy operating lymphatic system, because it protects us from disease and further inflammation by draining our system; keeping it clean if you will. When the lymphatic system is clogged, toxins build up causing further inflammation, disease and also infections.

When we experience an auto-immune disorder, we are also experiencing a build-up of lymphatic fluid, an excess from tissues and organs, that cannot drain properly which causes swelling. The lymphatic system, a network of vessels, is also responsible for circulating white blood cells to fight infection, via the spleen and lymph nodes. Since the lymphatic system is part of the immune system, there is a disconnect when the immune system is compromised from an auto-immune disorder. The immune system is designed to protect the body and keep it healthy by fighting off foreign invaders but in an auto-immune disease, it instead mistakenly or incorrectly recognizes healthy cells, self-antigens or autoantigens (normal proteins within the body) in your tissues, joints, organs, skin, bone, nerves, glands, blood vessels and even eyes as foreign and bad. The body's own T-cells (type of white blood cell) attack the perceived invaders causing much discomfort and tissue damage within. The discomfort of swelling, stiffness, warmth and pain can affect mobility greatly as well as causing a great amount of fatigue.

Since the immune system turns against the body it is designed to protect and since there then becomes a build-up of lymphatic fluid within, there needs to be a way to help release that build-up. Enter again the therapeutic tool, the Sanddune Stepper. Just by doing movements such as a deep squat hold on the Sanddune Stepper for 5-10 seconds, then rising up slowly and back down again slowly, creating that weightless feeling, it resets if you will, the Central Nervous System in such a way as to release build-up of lymphatic fluid. After the resetting position, the squat, quick movements up and down, in and out of the squat position, it engages the CNS, the lymphatic system and also the immune system in a feedback loop response with a rebound effect, helping to detoxify the lymphatic system and stimulate the immune system to respond properly.

The Sanddune Stepper is an incredible therapeutic tool helpful in so many aspects of health including recovery, strength, endurance, mobility and re-setting of the brain to respond correctly to stimuli; perfect for any age or ailment. If you can get one shortly after your brain injury to help you to recover and incorporate it in your physical and vestibular therapy sessions, you will be much farther ahead on your road to recovery. If indeed you do experience and auto-immune disorder or Fibromyalgia, as well as any neurological disease, nervous system issues, or just want to improve balance, strength and mobility, look into this as the results are amazingly worth it!

The great part about this, besides the wonderful ability to regain connections lost, is the accessibility to be able to do this in the comfort of your own home for the fraction of the cost of neurofeedback visits elsewhere for therapy and with a better response as there has been a great deal of promise and positive results with this one tool; plus, it is extremely easy on the joints which is a huge benefit if you suffer from joint pain and arthritis. In fact, it is so good at its results that it is being placed in physical therapy offices as well as gyms, and other beneficial places of help for people in recovery and rehabilitation settings. I just love mine! It surely has helped me a great deal, more so than traditional physical therapy.

I highly recommend the Sanddune Stepper for its beneficial results and relief, ease, as well as compact ability as it is completely portable, which means you will want to take it with you and show your friends, or just get outside with it to enjoy some fresh air. They even thought of that convenience by throwing in a convenient carrying bag with handles. How perfect is that. You may even want to bring it to your next doctor's appointment and show them what they are missing—a drug free alternative that really works.

Balls

Anytime you can find tools to help engage your brain during exercise, the better. The variety can be endless really as you can use your imagination to utilize almost anything as a helpful additive to your exercise routine. One such item is a ball. So, let's talk balls.

Now I'm not talking about the slang term, although I'm sure that is coming to mind for some of you reading this, but actual balls ranging in many sizes, shapes and of course textures. There are big ones, little ones, smooth ones and knobby textured ones. The balls I am talking about are used for therapy that benefit motor skills, stability, athletic training and very importantly coordination.

There are balls you can squeeze for hand and grip strength as well as stress relief when things get too overwhelming. There are balls that bounce straight and balls that bounce off into unknown directions, and balls that take off into the air as if into infinity, such as beach balls. The idea is to track the movement of the balls as you try to retrieve them—not like a golden retriever but you get the idea. It can be challenging for your healing brain and also helps with proprioception.

Do you want some real challenging fun, try catching a beach ball on a windy day. Okay maybe not if that will only cause you to be frustrated. You will have to bring along that stress ball and squeeze hard.

You may want to try a game of tennis as it can be challenging at first but rewarding as well, as you not only track the movement of the ball with your eyes but also engage your lower extremities while trying to hit it with the racket as you move about the court. This is a therapy lesson all its own. It surely is stimulating to the vestibular system, for sure. Of course, if you are not quite ready or stable on your feet, caution is advised as we do not want you to trip over your own feet. But, if you are up for it, then go for it as it is a lot of fun and great exercise to boot. You may notice using muscles you have long forgotten about as you "stop short" to hit that ball.

Weighted balls are perfect for athletic training and toning as they add just that little bit of density to your routine of exercise movements. They are easy to hold onto with both hands and work great for additional weight added to squats, lunges and also abdominal crunches. When you are more seasoned and comfortable with a particular weight, and I am talking lighter in this reference, you can even play around with catching them. However, please make sure you are capable of catching the weight as it will feel heavier with the applied force of movement in the air as well as the gravity as it descends to land into your hands. Also, watch it doesn't land on your toes because that would hurt for sure. Everyone knows that no matter how little or light something is, when it lands on your toe, suddenly it weighs a ton. Ouch!

In addition to smooth stability balls for balance, there are also available textured stability balls that add for a tactile sensation as they help activate and strengthen the body's core (mid-section of the body containing the body's stabilizing muscles) while increasing balance and stability.

Textured balls also come in small sizes that are perfect for tracking eye movements and body coordination as you try to catch them, not knowing in which direction it will go. They will ultimately challenge both your brain and your brawn.

Okay back to the hand-held stress balls that you can squeeze not only to relieve stress and anxiety but also develop strength and maintain hand/finger mobility. This involves a great and very helpful as well as appreciated little story. My son came home from school the other day and told me he wanted to buy some slime, (typical of a young boy I thought). So, his big sister, my younger daughter, graciously took him to buy some. To my surprise and surprising delight, as I do not like the feel of slime very much, I was impressed. He had me hold open a balloon, which we already had, so he can fill it with the slime. Hmmmm.... Well, besides the challenge of holding the balloon open while my fingers were locking into position, that slime filled balloon was just what I needed, though it was exactly what he wanted. We tied it and viola—a home-made squeeze ball at a very economical price; the slime was a buck at the local dollar store. Now, that's a value!

I was just so impressed by this I told him, "This is going in the book!", to his delight. What came out of my mouth next, I thought I would never say, "We have to go the store to buy more slime!" Yeah! Wonder if the neighbors heard my excitement. Mom of the year for that comment. Somehow squeezing that gooey substance through the balloon was "A-OK". In fact, it made my hands and fingers, that were locking, feel great! It is so easy on the joints! Who would have thought? A bright boy just wanting to make something cool. Try it. I can only imagine what the store clerk will say when I come to the counter, thrilled, with a bunch of slime. It's going to be priceless!

Memory **G**ames

Memory games are very useful in helping with memory challenges as well as supporting cognitive function. If we've suffered a brain injury, we may very well know what it is like to have difficulty with our memory, whether it be short or long-term or even both. We may have trouble concentrating still. If we are experiencing new or even never-ending memory challenges and brain fog due to our new auto-immune disorder or even Fibromyalgia, memory games can support us in ways that help us make those new connections in trying to remember. We can actually play memory games by having cards flipped over and mixed up, while we try to remember the matches that are hidden. We can walk into a room, take a brief look around, walk out again, then try to recall what we have seen. We can set things to music or play songs, trying to remember the lyrics, even if we have made them uniquely our own.

Names are often a hard thing to remember when we meet somebody new but when we repeat their name back to the person, it engages our auditory senses as well as sight. Attaching little clues or acronyms to names, things, or anything we try to remember adds another helpful element as we may feel like a detective solving a huge case. We may also want to try placing something out of its normal place, for yet another clue to our never-ending puzzle game, to act as a purposeful trigger, to engage our brain.

We can also do some little things like writing it down—everything if we need to. We can color code for categories of what we would like to remember. Often times we find ourselves repeating things over and over again in attempts to remember what we do not want to forget. With a little explaining on our part, as people can get annoyed by our repetition very easily, and a little understanding on their part, as to why we are repeating, will make for a more relaxing environment.

We can use bells, bracelets, colors, sounds, even fluorescent markers with sticky notes all around, or whatever we like and can come up with to make our own memory game. We can get very creative to think and to engage our brain, of our own ways to help aid in increasing our memory as well as our creativity.

Additionally, timers and alarms are perfect to set for just about anything we would like to remember, and when they go off, we can be amazed at how we may struggle at what they are even ringing for. It is that "Oh yeah!" moment. What is especially nice is that they are portable, even as close and convenient as our cells phones; plus, they can come with us wherever we may wander off to.

There are just so many helpful alternatives to conventional therapies and medicine that are available and can be potentially very positive with regards to a healing prognosis. We should never give up, rather look for what does help. We do not have to live in despair when the doctor tells us that he/she does not know what else to do, or that we've met a plateau, therefore cannot expect any further healing. There is always a way if you are still alive and breathing to improve! We have to believe it in our heart of hearts. We have to hold onto hope when all others have given up on us.

How many times have you heard stories where a doctor said someone will never walk again—but they did. They defied logic. Why? Because faith is not logical. It is a willingness to believe and to pursue hope. The nature of faith is that it must be tested, it must be tried because it is something that although we may not currently see, yet we believe anyway. Faith is the substance of things hoped for, for things we don't yet see, but the evidence that they can still come; if we only just believe.

Prayer

An additional tool to end this chapter is the ever-ready ability to pray, anytime and anywhere. Praying with hopeful purpose and intent in mind helps engage our thought processes for a better today, tomorrow and a better "right now". We are never really alone in this or anything else as we do have a helper, a constant friend that is closer than any brother, as He will not ever leave nor forsake us; He will give us the comfort, the strength, and the resources we need to get through. We can pray with a thankful heart for all the blessings we do have, and we may find a blessing coming through our pain as well. We may have tears for a night, or two, but joy always comes through. Our pain will not be wasted! Jesus holds all our tears. Our mourning can turn into a morning with a new dawn; a spark of light through our darkness.

We will often find that when we just "let go" and "let God" that we will have peace right in the middle of our storm as He works out the details on what to do next and where to go—the help coming our way and the healing process through it all. We are living in a fallen world full of fallen people that let us down, with fallen ailments, diseases, and challenges of every kind. But we are not alone, ever! Remember that! I've seen it and experienced it first hand so many times to ever deny God's presence. If you need Him, just call out to Him; He's right there waiting to help you.

You have not been brought this far to just give up and quit now! No! You must endure, and you must persevere. We all must. We must all have that fighting spirit to keep going. We must fight, not against ourselves, but against that status quo of the limits placed on us. Only God knows how far we can go and how much we can heal, to get back some normality and even experience a blessing out of it.

This injury and all that comes about from it may very well be our biggest giant we have ever faced in life yet. So, we cannot afford to be fearful and live in fear or worry of our circumstances. We really do need to rise above by being strong in our adversity and having good courage. We can be like Joshua and Caleb seeking out the promised land only to find giants living among the land. Most of the scouts with them that day fled in fear, falsely thinking they could not conquer them. However, Joshua and Caleb were most brave and knew that if they were brought to it, that God would bring them through it. They believed they could conquer their giants, and they did! They did not let any giant steal from them that which was promised.

The same goes for King David when he came to the face of his giant Goliath; huge and terrifying. Goliath surely attempted to place fear into David's heart as he tried to intimidate, disdain and frighten him with his armour and heavy weaponry. But David did not let it get to him, or his mission to defeat him. All David had was five smooth stones, one for Goliath and one for each of his brothers, and a whole lot of hope. He had unwavering faith and a fighting spirit to stand up and keep going in the midst of facing his giant. He had faith in a higher power that God was not just going to leave him there. No, he knew that if God brought him that far that he would be with him still in the battle in the valley. David ran towards his giant and defeated him! Can we fully understand that? Most of us would recoil and run the other way. We hide when things go wrong, when life gets tough and deals us some pretty rotten apples. We can learn a lot from these stories, from this history lesson. We can learn that it takes courage, moxy, and tenacity to not give up but rather just keep going.

Though this may be your biggest giant yet, you can beat it. You do not have to let it rob you any longer. It does not have to steal your joy. You can get that hope back again. You can try new therapies and tools to help. You can have hope in the middle of your storm, your valley, your trial; right in front of your giant. You can become healthier instead of sicker by looking into natural ways of healing that will invigorate your body and your spirit. You can be uplifted rather than being crushed down. You can endure, and you can persevere. You can be a warrior that fought and is still fighting a tough battle! How or why? Because you've been given grace. For that, you can once again smile as you look forward to a dream in your future; a dream that is yours alone to chase after and accomplish.

Now may the Lord of peace himself give you
his peace at all times and in every situation.
The Lord be with you all.
2 Thessalonians 3:16 NLT

"O Lord, by these things men live, And in all
these is the life of my spirit; O restore me to
health and let me live!
Isaiah 38:16 NASB

And he said unto her, Daughter, be of good
comfort: thy faith hath made thee whole; go in
peace.
Luke 8:48 KJV

For I can do everything through Christ, who gives me strength.
Philippians 4:13 NLT

If you do not yet know Jesus Christ as your own personal Savior and would like to, here is a sample prayer on the following page. The main thing to remember is not so much the words you say, but the meaning and sincerity from your heart, knowing and realizing that since all of us have sinned and fall short, (this is a fallen world and we all have done wrong-against a Holy God) that you too are a sinner. But, also know that Jesus died in yours and my place, because He loves us that much, (to take our punishment upon Himself), and rose again. We now need to turn from our sins as well as repent of our sins and believe in Christ as our own personal Savior to be saved. We can go to Him and talk to Him any time, anywhere. It was God Himself that came down to save us on that cross at Calvary, so we can be free from the power of sin and death, having peace instead, along with an eternity of peace in paradise; life everlasting.

Just turn your heart towards Jesus and pray to receive Him and His free gift of salvation; His forgiveness for your sins by faith. Through His forgiveness, His arms will lift you and His blood will cleanse you. Jesus' love will change you. Remember, God's grace and mercy is new every morning and His love is everlasting.

Jesus replied to the thief on the cross next to Him, that believed in Him...

Jesus answered him, "Truly I tell you, today you will be with me in paradise." Luke 23:43 NIV

Salvation Prayer

Dear Lord, I know that I am a sinner, and I ask for your forgiveness. I believe Jesus Christ died for my sins and rose from the dead. I accept your free gift of Salvation and the forgiveness of my sins. I trust and follow you as my Lord and Savior. Lord Jesus come into my heart, guide my life and help me to do your will. Thank you for reaching out to me, to save me. In Jesus name, I pray. Amen.

Therefore if any man be in Christ, he is a new creature: old things are passed away; behold, all things are become new.
2Corinthians 5:17 KJV

This means that anyone who belongs to Christ has become a new person. The old life is gone; a new life has begun!
2Corinthians 5:17 NLT

Helpful Links

Ganoderma (Reishi Mushroom) Coffee...Beverages & Nutraceuticals—Click on the "Beverage" Tab for Ganoderma Coffee:
http://rockmanjohnson.successbyhealth.com/

Moringa Oleifera—
http://www.greenvirginproducts.com?aff=112

Sanddune Stepper Therapy Tool—Click on The "News" Tab for Therapeutic Benefits:
http://www.sanddunestepper.com/

Notes

Get the Stats on Traumatic Brain Injury in the Unites States, https://www.cdc.gov/traumaticbraininjury/pdf/bluebook_factsheet-a.pdf

What is Arnica Montana? http://www.arnicare.com/about/arnica-montana/

What is Natural Vanilla Flavor, Natural Force, https://naturalforce.com/nutrition/natural-vanilla-flavor/

Cocaine: A Brief History, The Truth About Cocaine, Foundation for a Drug-Free World, https://www.drugfreeworld.org/drugfacts/cocaine/a-short-history.html

Poppy Plant, The Editors of Encyclopaedia Britannica, https://www.britannica.com/plant/poppy

During Learning, Neurons Deep in Brain Engage in a Surprising Level of Activity, Princeton University, Science News, https://www.sciencedaily.com/releases/2017/03/170321092731.htm

Prolactin, Wikipedia The Free Encyclopedia, https://en.wikipedia.org/wiki/Prolactin

Dopamine, Wikipedia The Free Encyclopedia, https://en.wikipedia.org/wiki/Dopamine

Lienard Sarah, What Is the Dopamine Diet? BBC Good Food, https://www.bbcgoodfood.com/howto/guide/what-dopamine-diet

Prolactin, You and Your Hormones, An Education Resource for the Society of Endocrinology, http://www.yourhormones.info/hormones/prolactin/

What is Auto-immune Disease? Sharecare, https://www.sharecare.com/health/immune-lymphatic-system-disorders/what-is-an-autoimmune-disease

Antinuclear Antibodies (ANA), American College of Rheumatology, https://www.rheumatology.org/I-Am-A/Patient-Caregiver/Diseases-Conditions/Antinuclear-Antibodies-ANA

Home Remedies for Candida, Top 10 Home Remedies, https://www.top10homeremedies.com/home-remedies/home-remedies-candida.html

9 Candida Symptoms & 3 Steps to Treat Them, Dr. Axe Food is Medicine, https://draxe.com/candida-symptoms/

How a Traumatic Brain Injury Can Lead to Fibromyalgia, Fibromyalgia Treating, http://www.fibromyalgiatreating.com/brain-injury-fibromyalgia/

Marshall Rick, The Origins of 11 Famous Star Trek Lines, http://mentalfloss.com/article/50607/origins-11-famous-star-trek-lines

The Changeling, Star Trek Transcripts, http://www.chakoteya.net/StarTrek/37.htm

CBD For Fibromyalgia, Healthline, https://www.healthline.com/health/cbd-for-fibromyalgia

Gabapentin, WebMD, https://www.webmd.com/drugs/2/drug-14208-8217/gabapentin-oral/gabapentin-oral/details

The Doctors Staff, The Dangers of Prescription Medication Gabapentin, The Doctors, https://www.thedoctorstv.com/articles/4421-the-dangers-of-prescription-medication-gabapentin

Bloom Josh, Neurontin: Overhyped and Underwhelming, American Council on Science and Health, https://www.acsh.org/news/2017/12/26/neurontin-over-hyped-and-underwhelming-12242

Tsai Alexander C., Gabapentin, Opioids, and the Risk of Opioid-Related Death: A Population-Based Nested Case-Control Study, NCBI PubMed, https://www.ncbi.nlm.nih.gov/pmc/articles/PMC5626029/

Cymbalta, WebMD, https://www.webmd.com/drugs/2/drug-91491/cymbalta-oral/details

St. John's Wort For Treating Depression, WebMD, https://www.webmd.com/drugs/2/drug-91491/cymbalta-oral/details

Fibromyalgia, Mayo Clinic, https://www.mayoclinic.org/diseases-conditions/fibromyalgia/symptoms-causes/syc-20354780

Lockhart Emily, The 10 Most Common Signs of Fibromyalgia, Active Beat, https://www.activebeat.co/your-health/the-10-most-common-signs-of-fibromyalgia/10/

Dellwo Adrienne, Is Fibromyalgia an Auto-immune Disease?, Very Well Health, https://www.verywellhealth.com/is-fibromyalgia-an-autoimmune-disease-716148

Rana M G MD, Fibromyalgia Mystery Finally Solved! Researchers Finally Find Main Source of Pain, https://fibromyalgiaresources.com/fibromyalgia-mystery-blood-vessels/

Vitality 101 with Dr. T, Overview of CFS and Fibromyalgia, CFS & Fibromyalgia, http://www.vitality101.com/cfs-and-fibromyalgia-overview

Passion Flower For Hot Flashes, Depression and Better Sleep, Dr. Axe Food is Medicine, https://draxe.com/passion-flower/

Rose Amy, Yikes! High Fructose Corn Syrup Health Risks, Earths Friends, https://www.earthsfriends.com/high-fructose-corn-syrup-health-risks/

Improving Proprioception and Ankle Strategy With New Balance Pad, EnsignTherapy.com, http://ensigntherapy.com/improving-proprioception-ankle-strategy-new-balance-pad/

Nevares Alana M. MD, Larner Robert MD, Mixed Connective Tissue Disease, Merck Manual Consumer Version, https://www.merckmanuals.com/home/bone,-joint,-and-muscle-disorders/autoimmune-disorders-of-connective-tissue/mixed-connective-tissue-disease-mctd

These 7 Ways To Help Autoimmune Disorders Make A Difference!, NSI Stem Cell, https://nsistemcell.com/7-ways-to-help-autoimmune-disorders/

What is a Naturopathic Doctor? Naturopathic Physicians: Natural Medicine. Real Solutions. https://www.naturopathic.org/content.asp?contentid=60

Johnson, C. Rae, Traumatic Brain Injury: TBI & Post-Concussion Syndrome: PCS Do's & Don'ts A Personal Journey

Andrews, Ryan, All About Lectins: Here's What You Need to Know, What Are Lectins? Precision Nutrition, https://www.precisionnutrition.com/all-about-lectins

Lectins: The Anti-nutrient, Body Ecology, https://bodyecology.com/articles/lectins-the-anti-nutrient

Leaky Gut Syndrome: What Is It?, WebMD, https://www.webmd.com/digestive-disorders/features/leaky-gut-syndrome#1

Ghrelin, Wikipedia, https://en.wikipedia.org/wiki/Ghrelin

Leptin, Wikipedia, https://en.wikipedia.org/wiki/Leptin

23 Foods that Increase Leptin Sensitivity, MedLicker, https://medlicker.com/1038-foods-that-increase-leptin-sensitivity

Dr. Mercola, Coconut Oil for Crohn's, Dr. Mercola, https://articles.mercola.com/sites/articles/archive/2017/07/10/coconut-oil-for-crohns.aspx

Too Much Sugar is Linked to Inflammation, Healthline, https://www.healthline.com/nutrition/sugar-and-inflammation

8 Food Ingredients That Cause Inflammation, Arthritis Foundation, https://www.arthritis.org/living-with-

arthritis/arthritis-diet/foods-to-avoid-limit/food-ingredients-and-inflammation-8.php

Cocao Nibs: Superfood That Boosts Energy and Burns Fat, Dr. Axe Food is Medicine, https://draxe.com/cacao-nibs/

Godinez Brenda, 10 Powerful Benefits of Drinking Moringa Every day, Mind Body Green, https://www.mindbodygreen.com/0-22401/10-powerful-benefits-of-drinking-moringa-every-day.html

The Vagus Nerve, Teach Me Anatomy, http://teachmeanatomy.info/head/cranial-nerves/vagus-nerve-cn-x/

3 Ways Moringa Benefits Arthritis (Science Baked), Natural Arthritis Treatments, https://www.naturalarthritistreatments.net/arthritis-in-general/3-ways-moringa-benefits-in-arthritis-science-backed

Bone Broth Benefits for Digestion, Arthritis and Cellulite, Dr. Axe Food is Medicine, https://draxe.com/the-healing-power-of-bone-broth-for-digestion-arthritis-and-cellulite/

10 Healthiest Fermented Foods & Vegetables, Dr. Axe Food is Medicine, https://draxe.com/fermented-foods/

Omega-3 Benefits, Including for Heart and Mental Health, Dr. Axe Food is Medicine, https://draxe.com/omega-3-benefits-plus-top-10-omega-3-foods-list/

Schisandra Benefits Adrenals & Liver Detox, Dr. Axe Food is Medicine, https://draxe.com/schisandra/

Reishi Mushroom: Helps Fight Cancer , Boost Immunity, and Improve Liver Detox, Reishi Mushroom, Dr. Axe Food is Medicine, https://draxe.com/food-category/reishi-mushroom/

Dr. Edward Group DC, NP, DACBN, DCBCN, DABFM, Chaga Mushroom: The Immune Boosting Superfood, Global Healing Center, Live Healthy, https://www.globalhealingcenter.com/natural-health/chaga-mushroom-the-immune-boosting-superfood/

Schizandra Berry...Want Help for Stress and Adrenal Fatigue, Natural Health and Healing 4U.com https://www.natural-health-and-healing-4u.com/schizandra-berry.html

7 Proven Chlorella Benefits (#2 is Best), Dr. Axe Food is Medicine, https://draxe.com/7-proven-chlorella-benefits-side-effects/

Top 10 Inflammation-Fighting Foods, Body Building.com, https://www.bodybuilding.com/content/top-10-inflammation-fighting-foods.html

Gabric Andrea, Nutritional Benefits of the Strawberry, WebMD, https://www.webmd.com/diet/features/nutritional-benefits-of-the-strawberry

You Can Eat, Healthline, https://www.healthline.com/nutrition/13-anti-inflammatory-foods

Avocado, Healthline, https://www.healthline.com/nutrition/12-proven-benefits-of-avocado

Hemp Seed Nutrition, Hemp Basics, https://www.hempbasics.com/shop/hemp-seed-nutrition

Can Hemp Repair DNA, Ergogenics, http://www.ergogenicsnutrition.com/blog/hemp-can-repair-dna/

Goji Berry Benefits: Antioxidant & Anti-inflammatory Superfruit, Dr. Axe Food is Medicine, https://draxe.com/goji-berry-benefits/

Eleuthero Root (Siberian Ginseng) an Underrated Adaptogen, Medicinal Herbals, https://medicinalherbals.net/eleuthero-root-siberian-ginseng-underrated-adaptogen/

Phytosterols: Sterols & Stanols, Cleveland Clinic, https://my.clevelandclinic.org/health/articles/17368-phytosterols-sterols--stanols

Magin Meg, Sinhah Rebecca, Fincher Kelly, Inflammation and Vitamin D: The Infection Connection, Inflammation Research, PubMed, NCBI,

https://www.ncbi.nlm.nih.gov/pmc/articles/PMC416
0567/

Largeman-Roth Frances, 10 Foods That Fight Inflammation, U.S. News Health, https://health.usnews.com/health-news/blogs/eat-run/2015/03/23/10-foods-that-fight-inflammation

Dr. Edward Group DC, NP, DACBN, DCBCN, DABFM, 6 Health Benefits of Quercetin, Global Healing Center, Live Healthy, https://www.globalhealingcenter.com/natural-health/health-benefits-of-quercetin/

11 Ashwagandha Benefits for the Brain, Thyroid, & Even Muscles (!), Dr. Axe Food is Medicine, https://draxe.com/ashwagandha-benefits/

James Kayla, 13 Benefits of Drinking Kombucha Everyday, Natural Food Series, https://www.naturalfoodseries.com/13-benefits-drinking-kombucha-every-day/

N Levin-Agmon, E Theodor, RM Segal, Y Shoenfeld, Vitamin D in Systemic and Organ Specific Autoimmune Diseases, PubMed, NCBI, https://www.ncbi.nlm.nih.gov/pubmed/23238772

Godman Heidi, Harvard Health Letter, Regular Exercise Changes the Brain to Improve Memory and Thinking Skills, Harvard Health Blog, https://www.health.harvard.edu/blog/regular-exercise-changes-brain-improve-memory-thinking-skills-201404097110

Probiotics May Help Boost Mood and Cognitive Function, Healthbeat, Harvard Health Publishing Harvard Medical School, https://www.health.harvard.edu/mind-and-mood/probiotics-may-help-boost-mood-and-cognitive-function

5-HTP, Vitamins and Supplements, Web MD, https://www.webmd.com/vitamins/ai/ingredientmono-794/5-htp

McIntosh James, What is Serotonin and What Does it Do?, Medical News Today, https://www.medicalnewstoday.com/kc/serotonin-facts-232248

Chocolate & Dopamine, Healthy Eating, SF Gate, http://healthyeating.sfgate.com/chocolate-dopamine-3660.html

Collins Karen, MS, RD, CDN, We Hear So Much About Antioxidant Compounds in Chocolate. What About Cocoa and Chocolate Milk? AICR Health Talk, American Institute for Cancer Research, http://www.aicr.org/press/health-features/health-talk/2013/06june2013/cocoa-chocolate-antioxidants.html

8 Food Ingredients that Cause Inflammation, Arthritis Foundation, https://www.arthritis.org/living-with-arthritis/arthritis-diet/foods-to-avoid-limit/food-ingredients-and-inflammation-11.php

What Are the Possible Side-effects of Oral Steroids, Medicine Net, https://www.medicinenet.com/steroids_to_treat_art hritis/article.htm#what_are_the_possible_side_effec ts_of_oral_steroids

Mayo Clinic Staff, Prednisone and Other Corticosteroids, Mayo Clinic, https://www.mayoclinic.org/steroids/art-20045692

Denoon J Daniel, Why Steroids Are Bad for You, WebMD, https://www.webmd.com/fitness-exercise/news/20050316/why-steroids-are-bad-for-you#1

Biologics: Benefits and Risks, Arthritis Foundation, https://www.arthritis.org/living-with-arthritis/treatments/medication/drug-types/biologics/risks-benefits.php

Stone Kathlyn, Top 10 Biologic Drugs in the Unites States, The Balance, https://www.thebalance.com/top-biologic-drugs-2663233

Bowden Jonny, Ph.D., C.N.S., SAMe, The Most Effective Natural Cures on Earth

Bowden Jonny, Ph.D., C.N.S., Arnica for Muscle Pain and Inflammation, The Most Effective Natural Cures on Earth

Fibromyalgia Has Central Nervous System Origins, American Pain Society, http://americanpainsociety.org/about-us/press-room/fibromyalgia-clauw

Fibromyalgia Has Central Nervous System Origins, Science News, Science Daily, https://www.sciencedaily.com/releases/2015/05/150517071813.htm

What Are Musculoskeletal Disorders?, Musculoskeletal Disorders, Health Line, https://www.healthline.com/health/musculoskeletal-disorders

Nociceptor, Wikipedia, https://en.wikipedia.org/wiki/Nociceptor

7 Ways Cherry Juice Benefits Us, Healthline, https://www.healthline.com/health/food-nutrition/ways-cherry-juice-benefits-you#1

Lila Mary Ann, Anthocyanins and Human Health: As In Vitro Investigative Approach, Journal of Biomedicine and Biotechnology, PMC US National Library of Medicine National Institutes of Health, NCBI, https://www.ncbi.nlm.nih.gov/pmc/articles/PMC1082894/

Marijuana, Healthy Horns University Health Services, https://www.healthyhorns.utexas.edu/marijuana.html

Rough Lisa, Your Dog, Cat or Other Animal Ate High THC Cannibis: What To Do, Cannibis 101, Leafly, https://www.leafly.com/news/cannabis-101/animals-eating-thc-cannabis

Endocannabinoid System, Wikipedia, https://en.wikipedia.org/wiki/Endocannabinoid_system

Moody Liz, CBD is the Best Anti-inflammatory, Anti-cancer, Anti-anxiety, Superfood You're Not Eating, Functional Food, MBG Food, https://www.mindbodygreen.com/articles/what-are-the-effects-of-cbd

12 Turmeric Benefits That Rival Medications, Dr. Axe Food is Medicine, https://draxe.com/turmeric-benefits/

Turmeric Dosage for Pain Relief, Turmeric for Health, https://www.turmericforhealth.com/turmeric-dosage/turmeric-dosage-for-pain-relief

What is Frankincense Good For? 8 + Essential Oil Uses & Benefits for Healing, Dr. Axe Food is Medicine, https://draxe.com/what-is-frankincense/

Baikerikar Shruti, Can Evening Primrose Oil Help in Peripheral Neuropathy?, Salubrainous, https://www.salubrainous.com/evening-primrose-oil-for-neuropathy/

Salt II William B. MD, Rost S. Natalia MD, What is the Limbic System of the Brain, Share Care, https://www.sharecare.com/health/functions-of-the-brain/what-is-limbic-system-brain

Fibromyalgia, Auto-Immune Disease, The Neuroscience Team, http://theneuroscienceteam.com/fibromyalgia-auto-immune-disease/

Amygdala, Science daily, https://www.sciencedaily.com/terms/amygdala.htm

VanSistine Thomas K. MD, Fibromyalgia: Aerobic Fitness for Fibromyalgia, Spine-Health, https://www.spine-health.com/conditions/fibromyalgia/fibromyalgia-aerobic-fitness-fibromyalgia

Exercise and Depression, WebMD, https://www.webmd.com/depression/guide/exercise-depression#1

Top 10 Health Benefits of Stretching, Health Fitness Revolution, http://www.healthfitnessrevolution.com/top-10-health-benefits-of-stretching/

Sanddune Stepper, http://www.sanddunestepper.com

Webb G. Wanda PhD., CCC-SLP Neurology for Speech Language Pathologist (sixth edition), 2017, Sherrington's Scheme, Neurosensory Organization, Science Direct, https://www.sciencedirect.com/topics/neuroscience/interoceptor

Russin John Dr., Advanced Strength Training for the Feet, https://drjohnrusin.com/advanced-strength-training-for-feet/

Red Light Therapy Benefits, Research and Mechanism of Action, Dr. Axe Food is Medicine, https://draxe.com/red-light-therapy/

www.ingramcontent.com/pod-product-compliance
Lightning Source LLC
Chambersburg PA
CBHW022247290526
45785CB00015B/385